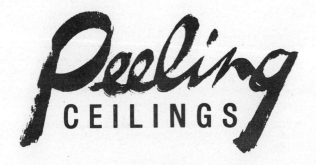

CEILINGS

500 <u>more</u>
Household Hints You Wanted to Know

by
Harris Mitchell

New questions and answers from
Canada's best-known authority on
home maintenance and improvement.

With more than 1,000 cross-referenced index listings.

 Published by Consumers' Association of Canada

A Harris Mitchell Book

Published by: Consumers' Association of Canada
Box 9300
Ottawa, Ontario, K1G 3T9

Canadian Cataloguing in Publication Data

Mitchell, Harris, 1916-
Peeling ceilings: 500 more household hints you wanted to know

Includes index.
ISBN 0-919005-02-0

1. Repairing—Amateurs' manuals. 2. Dwellings—Maintenance and
repair—Amateurs' manuals. I. Consumers' Association of Canada
II. Title.

TH4817.3.M48 1987   643'.7   C87-090316-0

ABOUT THE AUTHOR

As a home magazine editor and writer, Harris Mitchell has been dealing with house problems for more than 30 years. During this time, he has written hundreds of feature articles covering almost every aspect of home ownership and maintenance, and has appeared frequently on radio and TV as an authority on household problems.

He began writing his popular question-and-answer column, YOU WANTED TO KNOW, while editor of Western Homes & Living magazine in Vancouver, and continued the column when he became editor of Canadian Homes magazine, and later homes editor of Today magazine. Fourteen years ago, he started writing a syndicated weekly newspaper column that now appears in leading papers from Saint John to Vancouver. He receives, and answers, more than 3,000 questions a year from readers.

A book based on the column has gone through several editions, over 300,000 of which have been sold to date–a Canadian best-seller. The last edition, 1200 HOUSEHOLD HINTS YOU WANTED TO KNOW, also released simply as YOU WANTED TO KNOW, was published in 1982. The present book, PEELING CEILINGS, contains the answers to more than 500 new questions that have appeared in the newspaper column since the last book was published.

Harris Mitchell's other books include Canadian Homes Crafts, Easy Furniture Finishing, Plywood Projects, The Basement Book and How to Get More Heat for Your Fuel Dollar. He has also written several books for Canada Mortgage and Housing Corporation, and Energy, Mines and Resources, including How to Hire a Contractor, New Life for an Old House and Heating with Oil. He was also a consultant on all 36 volumes of the Time-Life Books series on home repair and improvement.

C O N T E N T S

AIR CONDITIONING

AIR CONDITIONER vs HUMIDIFIER

A couple of years ago we had a central air conditioner installed in our furnace. Since then our furnace humidifier has not been nearly as effective.

The air conditioner may have been installed incorrectly. A furnace humidifier is connected between the warm air duct and the cold air return duct, and the pressure difference between these two ducts when the fan is operating causes warm air to pass through the humidifier. However, if air conditioner coils are installed in the warm air duct *below* the humidifier, this will lower the pressure difference across it and therefore reduce the amount of air flowing through it. The remedy is to move the humidifier to a position between the cooling coils and the furnace.

AIR CONDITIONER CAUSES DAMPNESS INSIDE WALLS

We noticed a musty smell in the stairwell of our 2-storey home this summer, and I found that some of the gypsumboard panelling on the outside wall of the stairwell was damp and soft. I removed some of the panelling and discovered that the aluminum foil backing was dripping with water and the insulation behind it was soaking wet. What would cause this? The weather had been very hot and humid for a few weeks at that time and our central air conditioner had been working overtime to keep the house cool. Could this have anything to do with it?

It could indeed. Scientists at the National Research Council confirm that under certain conditions condensation can form inside the wall cavity of an air-conditioned house. This can happen when hot, humid outdoor air gets into the wall (which it does very easily from the outside) and then reaches the back of the cool inside wall. This is just the reverse of the winter condensation problem, when humid *indoor* air condenses on the *room* side of cold walls and windows. Actually, the condensation should only go as far as the vapor barrier - the aluminum foil, in your case - which should keep it from soaking into the gypsumboard, but it can still do a lot of damage to the insulation. In your case there must also be open seams, holes or other gaps in the vapor barrier that allow the condensation to get into the gypsumboard. The only way this can be repaired, incidentally, is to remove and replace damaged panelling.

Condensation like this may occur inside the walls of many air-conditioned homes, but it probably evaporates to the outside fairly quickly. And because the problem is usually hidden in the wall cavity, few people are ever aware of it. The only practical step that can be taken to prevent it, in any case, is to set the air conditioner thermostat to a higher temperature. Even an increase of a couple of degrees in room temperature would probably be enough to prevent most of the condensation that is occurring inside your walls during very humid summer weather.

CLAMMY AIR

We replaced our central air conditioner recently, and I insisted on getting a larger unit that would cool the house faster. Now the air in the house feels clammy, like a cool, damp basement. What causes this and how can I correct it?

Cooling is only half of the job an air conditioner does to make your house feel more comfortable in hot weather. It must also lower the humidity, and it does this by condensing moisture out of the air as it passes through the cooling coils inside the furnace. Achieving the right balance of cooling and dehumidification requires careful sizing of the equipment. Your former air conditioner was probably the right size. The larger one you have installed may cool the house quicker, but it does not run long enough to reduce the humidity. The result is a house filled with cool, clammy air that has a relative humidity close to 100%.

You could improve conditions with a couple of portable dehumidifiers, but this does not make much sense when you have central air conditioning. The proper remedy is to replace the outside compressor unit with one the same size that you had before - the one the installer wanted to put in in the first place, I would guess.

CLEANING A WINDOW AIR CONDITIONER

We have a window air conditioner that we use in our bedroom. It has given good service for several years, but I'm sure it must need cleaning or other attention by now. Is there anything I can do to keep it in good working condition?

It will do a better cooling job and last a lot longer if it is checked and cleaned every year before being put back in service. Remove the front of the air conditioner so you can reach the filter and the cooling coils behind it. Some front grilles are simply pried off; others are held on with a couple of screws. Plastic sponge filters can be cleaned by running warm water through them from the clean side to rinse out the dirt. Fibreglass filters should be replaced.

The cooling coils look like a small automobile radiator. Use the brush attachment on a vacuum cleaner to remove dust and lint from the fins. Bent fins can reduce the cooling capacity; straighten them gently with a broad putty knife or buy a special fin comb from an appliance parts store. The combs come in different sizes according to the number of fins per inch. (In some air conditioners, the cooling coils are covered with densely packed aluminum spines. Do not attempt to straighten these.)

There is a pan under the cooling coils that catches the condensation that drips from them during humid weather. The water passes through a drain pipe to another pan in the outside section of the unit, where it is evaporated. Use a piece of coathanger wire to clean the connecting drain pipe.

Remove the cover from the outside section to expose the compressor, fan motor and the condenser coils (which also look like a car radiator and do much the same job). These parts can be cleaned with a hose, but usually a vacuum cleaner is all you need. Straighten any bent fins on the condenser coil. Clean any deposit out of the drain pan.

Most fan motors have bearings that are permanently lubricated, but some require a few drops of SAE 20 oil once a year. Look for small oiling cups on each end of the motor – or check the owner's manual if you have one.

Rust spots on the cover should be rubbed down to bare metal with #100 silicon carbide paper, then covered with metal primer and matching enamel.

Check the power cord for damage. If the insulation has been cut, the plug casing is cracked, or the prongs are loose, disconnect the cord from the air conditioner (making a note of how the three wires are connected) and take it to an appliance parts store for a replacement.

DUCT SIZE FOR COOLING

We are thinking of installing central air conditioning this year, but have heard that our 5 in. furnace ducts are not large enough to handle the job. Is this correct?

It's true that a greater volume of air is required for cooling than for heating, so larger ducts would be better. Few homes have them, however, and central air conditioning works pretty well, anyway. One thing you can do to improve it is put a 2-speed fan in the furnace and use a higher speed for cooling.

BASEMENTS

ADJUSTING A MAIN BEAM

The main beam that runs the length of the basement in our bungalow is held up by three adjustable posts. How do I adjust these?

You do not have to adjust them at all unless the floor has sagged and the doors no longer close properly. Raising the jackposts under the beam will correct these problems, but it must be done very slowly. Raise the centre post no more than 1/16 in. a day, and the other two posts somewhat less. Check to make sure they are not just lifting the beam off its end supports; if they are, keep wetting the beam with a sponge or spray to make it more flexible. It may not be possible to level the beam completely. Stop when the upstairs problems are corrected.

DAMP BASEMENT

Our basement is damp and cool during the summer months and we can't store anything down there without it getting musty. I've heard there is a solution that you soak a towel in and then hang it over a pail. Water will collect on the towel and drip in the pail. What is the name of this solution?

I'm afraid there's no such solution. You may be thinking of calcium chloride, a chemical that, in dry form, absorbs water from the air. (It is also used to melt ice on roads and sidewalks in winter.) Flakes of calcium chloride placed in a cloth bag and hung over a pail will draw water from the air. This is a slow and expensive way to do it, however. An electric dehumidifier is much more efficient, and a lot cheaper to operate.

EFFLORESCENCE

A white powder keeps coming up between the floor tiles in our basement, and some of the tiles are getting loose. I have to keep sweeping up the powder, and now I would like to lay carpet on the floor, which seems perfectly dry, but I want to eliminate this powder problem first. I'm told that the only way I can stop it is to pour two inches of concrete on top of the tiles. Is this true?

The white powder is efflorescence, caused by water seeping up through the concrete and bringing with it dissolved salts that are left on the surface when the water evaporates. The floor *is* damp, in other words, but the water evaporates before you notice it. Adding another layer of concrete won't do much good. Moisture will continue to seep up through this as long as there is insufficient drainage under the floor.

The only remedy is to improve the drainage. The easiest way to do this is to put a sump pump in the floor, but the best way is to have a drainage contractor excavate and lay drainage tile wherever it's needed, either inside or outside the basement walls. I don't recommend laying carpet until this is done.

FRAMING A BASEMENT WALL

I plan to insulate and panel my basement walls before the cold weather comes. Is there anything wrong with building the 2x4 frame wall on the floor, about half an inch shorter than the wall height, then lifting it into position and driving wood shims under the bottom to snug it under the ceiling joists, where it would be nailed in place? This would avoid having to drive nails into the concrete.

The idea of raising the frame wall into position is perfectly sound, and often done, but putting shims underneath will leave a large gap where warm, humid household air can circulate behind the insulated wall and condense on the cold concrete. This would wet the insulation, rot the wood, and perhaps run out under the wall and damage the floor.

A better procedure is to place the shims between the top of the frame wall and the ceiling joists. A bead of caulking compound applied to the floor under the bottom plate before the wall is raised will prevent any air leakage there and also help to anchor the frame in position.

LEAK IN WALL/FLOOR JOINT

Two or three times a year, water seeps into our basement through the crack where the floor joins the wall in one area. How can I seal this?

First you should check outside to see if groundwater is getting down the outside of the wall at that spot. The earth may have settled there, the eavestrough may be overflowing, or a downspout may be discharging directly on the ground. These are easily corrected.

The crack can be sealed from the inside by chipping it out and filling the cavity with one of the expanding hydraulic cements that are made for this job, such as Thoro Waterplug, Bondex Quick Plug, Poly Kwikplug and Set Plug. The only difficut part of the job is chipping out a ¾ in. square or undercut channel for the patching material. You can do this with a hammer and cold chisel, but it is a lot easier if you rent a power chisel. Remove all dust and concrete particles with a shop vacuum. Mix and apply the plug material according to the manufacturer's instructions. It will set in three to five minutes, so only mix as much as you can use in that time. Wet the channel, then press enough compound into it to fill it completely. Add more and smooth it with a 1½ in. putty knife or a square-ended trowel to create a 45 degree chamfer or bevel in the floor/wall joint.

BASEMENT SWIMMING POOL

We are thinking of installing an above-ground pool in our basement, which has a fairly high ceiling. Is this practical?

Assuming you will have four feet of water in the pool, which is about the least you need for swimming, this will exert a pressure of 248 pounds per square foot (1220 kg/m²) on the floor. A properly laid 4-in. thick concrete floor should be able to support four times that weight, but older homes (and some newer ones, too) sometimes have concrete floors that are thinner than this - occasionally much thinner - so I do not think it would be smart to take the risk of severe cracking. After all, a circular pool just 10 ft in diameter will weight nine tons.

A heated indoor swimming pool like this presents another problem. Even if it is covered when not in use it will add a considerable amount of moisture to the air in your home, and probably cause condensation, mildew, wood decay and other troubles associated with excessive humidity. Properly designed indoor swimming pools must use heavy-duty ventilating equipment to prevent such problems.

WALL CRACKED

We have a crack in our poured concrete foundation wall that leaks quite badly during wet weather. You have said that the best way to patch such a crack is from the outside, but the builder wants to inject an epoxy compound from the inside. Will this make a permanent repair?

Only if there is no further movement of the concrete wall at that point. This is unlikely, however, and I think it is much better to seal the crack from the outside with a flexible patch.

Cover the crack with a heavy coat of fibrated asphalt roofing cement extending at least 3 in. on both sides, then reinforce this with a 6 in. wide strip of fibreglass and let this dry for a couple of days before backfilling the excavation very carefully to avoid damaging the patch.

If the builder insists on doing it his way, ask for *written* assurance that he will repair the crack if it leaks again *any time in the future.*

WATERPROOFING WITHOUT DIGGING

We have had a problem with a wet basement for many years, but I've put off having someone dig down and repair the drain tile because of the cost and because we have a sidewalk, extensive foundation planting, and a concrete patio. I've seen ads for waterproofing treatments that require no digging. Do they really work? Are they guaranteed?

One system consists of pushing a long nozzle down the outside of the foundation wall and pumping in a thin slurry of bentonite, a collodial clay that is used for sealing oil wells and reservoirs. If the location of the basement leak can be determined, and if the bentonite can reach it, this method is often successful. It's certainly a lot cheaper than digging, but it doesn't always work. Most firms will come back and try again if the first application fails, but if other work is needed to cure the problem, they'll charge you for it.

Another method that avoids outside digging is to install a drainage ditch *inside* the house. This is done by cutting a trench about a foot wide through the basement floor just inside the wall and connecting it to the floor drain or a sump pump. Holes are drilled in the foundation wall to relieve outside water pressure and drainage pipe is laid in the trench. This is covered with gravel and topped with concrete to the original floor level. The process is more expensive than the bentonite treatment but cheaper than digging down outside the house, particularly where this would involve considerable reconstruction work, as in your case.

BRICK

CLEANING BRICK

My brick bungalow is 25 years old. The brick is smooth and in good condition, but the color has darkened and looks very dull. A lot of brick houses in the United States are painted, and I would like to know if you think this is a good idea in Canada.

I've seen a lot of painted brick houses here, too, but most of them look pretty tatty after a few years. Then comes the big job of removing all the loose paint and applying a new coat. This becomes a regular maintenance job that is both tedious and expensive. One of the main advantages of brick, surely, is that it requires very little maintenance.

A good cleaning will restore the original color and last a lot longer than a paint job. You can use one of the commercial masonry cleaners or a solution of one part muriatic acid to 10 parts water. Wear rubber gloves, protect your eyes, and be careful to keep the acid off skin and clothing. Wet the brick thoroughly and let the water sink in before applying the cleaning solution. Rinse off thoroughly with a hose.

Brick can also be cleaned with a high-pressure water spray. This may remove loose mortar but will not damage brick or solid mortar. The equipment is available from most tool rental stores.

DIRT MARKS ON BRICK WALL

Our eavestroughs overflowed last year and spattered dirt on the bottom of our brick walls. What is the best way to remove this?

Brush off as much of the dirt as you can when it is dry, then soak the bricks with water and use a scrubbing brush to apply a solution of one-quarter cup of dishwasher detergent to a gallon of water, or 50ml to 1 litre. Rinse off with a strong hose jet. Repeat if necessary.

REMOVING GRAFFITI FROM BRICKS

Young vandals used spray cans of different colored paints to "decorate" the brick walls of my house. Can I get this off myself, or is sandblasting the only remedy?

Sandblasting is not recommended because it cuts back the soft mortar joints, rounds off the edges of the bricks and removes the hard, protective surface that keeps out moisture. Chemical removers do a much better job when used in conjunction with a powerful water spray to blast the softened paint off the rough-textured bricks. Standard paint removers available at any hardware store will soften most paints, but a much cheaper and more effective paint remover for a brick wall is a strong lye solution you can make yourself. In a quart glass jar dissolve half of a 9½-ounce can of lye (available at any grocery store) in one pint (20 ounces) of water. In another container mix four heaping tablespoons of flour or corn starch with a pint of water, then pour this slowly into the lye solution, stirring constantly to make a smooth, thick paste.

(If you prefer metric measure, dissolve 130 grams of lye in 500ml of water in a 1 litre jar, then add another 500ml of water mixed with 100ml of flour or corn starch.)

This strong caustic mixture is a very effective paint remover, but it must be used carefully. Wear rubber gloves and protect your eyes with glasses. If any of the lye paste gets on your skin, wipe it off immediately with a wet cloth. Protect plants with a plastic drop sheet.

Use an old paint brush to apply a thick coat of the lye mixture on test areas of the different paints that were used. Leave for at least 45 minutes, then flush off the softened paint with a high-pressure water jet (around 1000psi). You can rent such spray-cleaning equipment from most tool rental stores.

Auto body lacquers and some metallic paints that are unaffected by the lye solution can be removed with lacquer thinner or one of the standard paint removers, but you will still have to use the high-pressure spray to blast off the softened paint.

If you find a spot where the paint cannot be removed entirely from the textured surface of the bricks, the best remedy is to cover it with an exterior latex paint tinted to match the bricks.

GREY SCUM ON BRICKS

I used a solution of muriatic acid to remove some mortar stains from a brick wall. Most of the mortar marks have gone but the area I treated is covered with a greyish-white haze that will not come off with the acid solution or anything else I have tried.

Sometimes called mortar scum, this is caused by using too strong a solution of acid or not applying it properly. You should not use a solution stronger than one part muriatic acid to 10 parts water (in spite of what it says on the labels of some brands). But it is also important to soak the bricks with water before the acid solution is applied, and to rinse them off thoroughly af-

terwards. Failure to follow these steps may leave a grey film of silicic acid on the bricks that can be very difficult to remove. The most effective solvent is hydrofluoric acid, the acid that dissolves glass, but this is very difficult to get and dangerous to use. Brick manufacturers suggest using a solution of one part vinegar to one part water. Soak the bricks with plain water, then apply this solution with a stiff brush or a coarse cloth, rubbing vigorously. If this does not work, you may be able to hide the stain with a solution of one part linseed oil to 10 parts petroleum solvent. But even if you do nothing, it will weather away in time.

REMOVING PAINT FROM BRICK

We recently bought a century-old brick house. Unfortunately some of the brick has been painted white, and we would like to remove this. Is sandblasting the only way to do it?

If you want to preserve a fine old brick house, sandblasting is definitely *not* the way to do it. This removes the hard, protective surface of the brick and some of the mortar, exposing the masonry to water penetration and subsequent deterioration.

Use a washable paint remover to soften the paint, and a strong water jet to remove it. (You can rent high pressure spray cleaning equipment from most tool rental shops.) If there are several coats of paint, you may have to use more than one application of paint remover.

SANDBLASTING OLD BRICK

What is your opinion of sandblasting old brickwork to restore it?

I don't know of a single authority on building restoration that recommends the use of sandblasting on old brickwork. It rounds the edges of the bricks and removes their hard, protective surface, leaving a soft, rough-textured face that catches dirt and absorbs water. Sandblasting also cuts back the soft mortar, producing recessed joints that catch rainwater. A report on brick cleaning methods published by the Building Research Division of the National Research Council says: "The effect of sandblasting on many buildings has been so harmful that the brickwork has been irreparably damaged . . . This method of cleaning should be avoided." Heritage Canada, responsible for the restoration and preservation of historic buildings, does not approve the use of sandblasting on old brickwork. Only steam or chemical treatment should be used.

SEALING POROUS BRICKWORK

The bricks and mortar on our 5-year-old house are very porous. What kind of a sealer can be applied to correct this?

The brick industry does not recommend the use of sealers, as a general rule, but sometimes they are the only remedy for a problem like this, which is really due to poor brickwork. The sealers are generally acrylic polymers that penetrate the suface and form a waterproof but vapor permeable layer on the face of the brick. Two brands that leave no discernable finish are Hydrozo (an industrial product) and Thompson's 101 Water Seal. Three brands that give the brickwork a wet look and darken the color are Thoroglaze, Watco Tile & Brick Sealer and Benjamin Moore's Silicone Acrylic Concrete Stain (clear). Apply as directed.

BRICK WALL FLAKING

We have a problem with the brick wall on the back of our bungalow. The brick seems to be flaking away in several places. Can you tell me what's causing this and what I can do about it?

This is called "spalling" and it's generally caused by moisture getting into the brick and freezing. Water may be leaking through cracks in the mortar joints; these should be chipped out about ¾ in. deep and then filled with new mortar applied with a narrow pointing tool. When the mortar begins to set, smooth it with a jointing tool or a short, curved length of copper pipe to make a tight, concave mortar joint that will shed water.

A leaking eavestrough or downspout is another possible source of the moisture. This is usually indicated by a white powder (see Efflorescence) on the surface of the bricks.

If the spalled brick is outside the bathroom or other area of the house where a lot of moisture is produced, the spalling is probably caused by humid air passing through the wall, where it condenses and freezes inside the bricks during cold weather. The best remedy is to put an exhaust fan in the room where the moisture originates. But you should also look for cracks where the humid air can leak out, such as along the bottom of the wall and around the window. Use a caulking compound or fibreglass wool to plug all such leaks.

WEEP HOLES IN BRICK VENEER

I would like to block the weep holes along the bottom of the brick veneer walls of our house to prevent cold air and bees from getting in. Someone has suggested that I put a short length of sash cord in the gap between the bricks to act like a wick, and then fill the gap with mortar. Is this a good idea?

I don't think so. I get a lot of letters asking about water leaking into the basement over the top of a foundation wall that supports brick veneer facing like this. There are many ways that rainwater can penetrate the brick wall and run down behind it, and weep holes are one of the measures required by the building code to keep this water from getting into the house.

A piece of sash cord is not going to provide nearly as much drainage as an open mortar joint, nor is it likely to be effective for very long. I do not think bees will be interested in your brick wall, and the amount of air that would get into the house through the weep holes is negligible. Water buildup behind the brick facing, on the other hand, could be a serious problem.

CARPETS

CANDLE WAX ON CARPET

During a recent power outage some candle wax dripped on our living room carpet. How can I remove this without harming the carpet?

Apply an ice cube to harden the wax, then break and scrape off as much as you can. Cover the spot with a folded paper towel and apply a hot iron. The towel will absorb the remaining wax as it melts. Repeat if necessary, then sponge the spot with a cloth moistened with a petroleum solvent such as Varsol or paint thinner.

FLOOR POLISH ON CARPET

While waxing the tile floor in our entrance hall the other day I spilled a bottle of acrylic floor polish on the adjoining carpet. I sponged off as much as I could but the carpet was still very stiff when it dried. Do you know of any way I can remove the acrylic polish from the carpet fibres?

A fairly strong solution of liquid household ammonia will break up the acrylic so it can be washed off. I suggest using one cup of ammonia to a quart of water. Sponge this on the carpet pile, let it stand for 10 minutes or so, then remove the granulated resin with a flow-through carpet cleaner rented from a supermarket or hardware store. Repeat if necessary.

This process will soak the carpet much more than is recommended, so remove the water as quickly as you can, using cloths, sponges or a water vacuum, then air-dry with plenty of ventilation. If only a relatively small area of the carpet is affected, there should not be enough shrinkage to cause any trouble.

GLUE ON CARPET

We have had what looks like an expensive accident. Contact cement was spilled on our wall-to-wall living room carpet. We cannot repair it by patching, because the color no longer matches the unused scraps of carpet we have available. Maybe I'm an optimist, but I'm hoping there is something that will dissolve contact cement without harming the carpet.

There is. Contact cement solvent can be purchased at any hardware store, and it will not harm nylon, wool, acrylic or polyester carpets.

HANGING A RUG

I was recently given a small Persian rug that I would like to hang on the wall in our living room. What is the best way to do this?

The best way that I know of is to nail a strip of "tackless" carpet edging to the wall and then hang the carpet on this. Tackless edging is a thin strip of wood with a row of closely spaced metal pins projecting at an angle, and it's used to anchor wall-to-wall carpeting around the perimeter of a room. It's available at any carpet supply store.

Cut a strip the width of the rug and nail it to the wall with 1½ in. ringed flooring nails centered over the studs. (To locate the studs, which are spaced 16 in. apart, tap the wall and listen for a solid sound, or use one of the magnetic stud locators.) The strip of tackless edging should be at the height you want the rug to be, and the pins should project upwards. You merely hang the rug on these pins.

RIPPLES ON THE CARPET

The wall-to-wall carpet in our living area, put down about 5 years ago, has developed ripples or waves. Is there anything we can do to correct this?

The carpet needs to be unhooked, stretched, trimmed and re-attached, and that is not a do-it-yourself job, I'm afraid. Call in an expert carpet-layer.

But if it keeps recurring it may be due to an inferior backing on the carpet. Carpet layers tell me that the new synthetic backing materials are causing far more stretching problems than jute ever did. The only remedy for this would be to replace the carpet.

RUGS THAT WALK

To protect the wall-to-wall broadloom in our living room I have added small area rugs in the main traffic routes. The problem I am having is that these keep wrinkling and moving sideways. I can't get them to stay flat where I put them. No one seems to know what is causing this or how to prevent it.

This happens because the pile of the broadloom carpet all slants in one direction, a result of the manufacturing process. When you walk on one of the area rugs the carpet pile is pressed down in this direction and acts like a ratchet, moving the rug along in that direction.

Many carpet stores sell a rubberized, open netting that can be laid under the area rug to prevent this happening. Or you can simply use a layer of polyester quilt batting, available at any fabric shop, to do the same thing.

RUST STAIN ON CARPET

How can I remove a rust stain from a white wool carpet?

Dissolve half a teaspoon of citric acid crystals (available from a druggist but also sold in grocery stores as "sour salt") in two ounces of water, add a quarter teaspoon of table salt and apply this to the rust stain with an eyedropper. Then hold a steam iron close to the carpet over the stain area. The rust stain should disappear in a few minutes. Rinse the spot by alternately dabbing it with a moist sponge and a dry towel.

Another method is to use a concentrated solution of oxalic acid crystals. These are available from a druggist (they may even have it on the shelves labelled as Rust Remover), or look in your grocery store for a household cleaning material called ZUD Rust Remover. You don't need to add salt to these, but steam will still speed the action.

CEILINGS

INSULATION VALUE OF SUSPENDED CEILING

Our house has a flat roof that is very diffi-cult to insulate. Would it do any good to put in a suspended ceiling with ½ in. softboard ceiling tiles? I understand these have some insulation value, and there would also be a 6 in. air space above them.

The insulation value of such a ceiling would be insignificant, I'm afraid. Air leakage through the suspended grid, and air currents behind it, would cancel the minimal benefit of the soft-board and the air space. Even if the suspended ceiling were perfectly sealed, the air space and the softboard would each add only .85 in insula-tion value, or R1.7 together. This is equivalent to less than half an inch of fibreglass batt.

The best remedy is to have insulation blown into the roof cavity. This can add up to R30 in insulation value.

LIFTING CEILING

We built our one-storey house four years ago, and every winter since then we have had a problem with gaps as large as half an inch opening up between the ceiling and the inside walls. It looks as if the ceiling is being lifted up, particularly down the centre of the house. In the spring the gaps close again as the ceiling appears to settle back to its proper place. What causes this and how can we correct it?

This problem was unknown until roof trusses replaced the traditional joist-and-rafter A-frame roof construction. Engineers have dis-covered that it is caused by differences in the moisture content of the "rafter" sections of the prefabricated roof truss, which is exposed to cold and very humid air, and the "joist" section, which is surrounded by insulation and there-fore remains relatively warm and dry. This causes the rafter sections to expand, and be-cause of the way a roof truss is constructed, it forces the joist section to arch upwards, taking the ceiling with it.

Although the problem is well understood, it is still quite rare, and apparently only happens if the truss is made of wood with a combination of unusual grain patterns. But when it does occur there is no practical way to stop it. The best remedy is to apply a strip of cove molding over the wall/ceiling crack, *nailing it only to the ceiling.* This will keep the crack hidden as it rides up and down with the lifting ceiling.

RECURRING CEILING CRACK

There is a crack in our dining room ceiling that reappears every year. I'm planning to paint the ceiling soon and would like to fix this persistent crack once and for all.

Recurring cracks like this are generally caused by the expansion and contraction of the house framework with seasonal changes in tempera-ture and humidity. The best remedy is to fill the crack and cover it with pliable patching mate-rial reinforced with fibreglass tape. Most hard-ware stores carry a product called Krack-Kote that comes in a kit that includes a roll of fi-breglass tape, the special patching compound and a spreading tool. This method won't work, however, if you have a textured ceiling.

WAVY CEILING

About a year ago we had a precut, packaged home put up on our lot in the cottage coun-try. The roof is supported on trusses that are spaced 24 in. apart, and the drywall ceiling panels are nailed to the underside of the trusses. Now we have noticed that the ceiling is wavy where the panels appear to have sagged between the trusses. Can you tell us what could cause this and how we can fix it without pulling the ceiling down?

Truss roofs are used on most houses these days, and 24 in. spacing is common. The most likely cause of your problem is the use of ⅜ in. gyp-sumboard panels on the ceiling. Nothing less than ½ in. should be used here, and ⅝ in. is bet-ter.

A contributing cause could be dampness in the attic due to the leakage of household air into this space and the lack of sufficient venti-lation to get rid of it. Check the attic for signs of condensation under the roof and dampness in the insulation. Measure the size of the vents in the roof and overhang. You should have one square foot of open vent area for every 300 ft² of ceiling.

If the insulation is damp, try to find where the humid air from the house is leaking into the attic and then seal these openings. Hot weather and good ventilation should dry out the insula-tion. Finally, apply another layer of gypsum-board to the ceiling using panel adhesive, then tape and fill the joints.

CERAMIC TILE

APPLYING CERAMIC FLOOR TILES

I am planning to have ceramic floor tiles (quarry tiles, actually) put down in our kitchen and entrance hall. Some people tell me these can be glued directly to the existing vinyl floor, which is firmly attached and in good condition. Others say the vinyl must be removed and a layer of cement mortar applied to the plywood subfloor to support the tiles properly and prevent the floor from bouncing and causing the joints to crack. This method is much more expensive. Which one should we use?

Laying the tiles on a bed of mortar is the traditional way to do it, but it is no longer the most common way. When ceramic tiles were made by hand and varied in thickness, the mortar would accept the different thicknesses and still provide a perfectly level floor. But this is not necessary with modern, machine-made tiles that are identical in thickness, and so they are now commonly laid with a flexible mastic adhesive that is simply applied with a notched trowel.

A bed of mortar will not prevent the floor from moving when it is walked on, in any case. If anything, the added weight will make the floor move even more. If the floor is too bouncy to support this kind of flooring, the remedy is to strengthen it by doubling the joists where necessary.

CLEANING SHOWER TILE GROUT

The white grout between the small ceramic tiles on the wall of our shower stall keeps getting dirty and is very hard to clean. Is there a special cleaner I should use?

Most of the black discoloration on bathroom tile grout is mildew mold, caused by the constant dampness. It can be removed with a strong solution of chlorine laundry bleach - one part to three parts water. Apply with a stiff brush.

Wiping the walls down with a towel after every shower will do much to prevent the mold from growing on the porous cement grout. It will also help if you use a small brush to paint the grout with silicone water repellent such as is sold for waterproofing leather shoes. The grout must be completely dry before this is applied, however. Any silicone that gets on the ceramic tile should be wiped off before it dries with a cloth moistened with petroleum solvent.

CERAMIC TILE COUNTERTOP

Our kitchen counters are plastic laminate and I would like to have them covered with ceramic tile, but a kitchen contractor tells me they break easily and are hard to clean. I've seen some beautiful kitchens with tile counters, however. Are they really practical?

I suspect that the contractor does not like ceramic tile because it is more difficult to apply than plastic laminate countertops. It is also more expensive, but ceramic tile is widely used on counters and I haven't heard any complaints. The choice is purely a matter of personal taste, I think.

Tile can be laid directly on the existing laminate as long as this is firmly attached, but the surface should be roughened with sandpaper first for a better bond. The tiles are applied using a mastic adhesive spread with a notched trowel. I don't know what color tile you plan to use, but I suggest using a dark-toned grout for easier cleaning.

CERAMIC TILE GROUT CRACKING

We removed the linoleum from our kitchen floor a few months ago and had ceramic tiles installed. Since then the colored cement grout between the tiles has been cracking and coming out. Where it is still in place, however, it seems very hard and is certainly difficult to remove. Why is it cracking?

I suspect this is due to the floor being too springy, a common problem when laying ceramic tiles on a wood frame floor. The best remedy is to strengthen the floor by nailing an additional joist to two or three of the existing joists. Loose grout will have to be removed and replaced with matching material.

WATERPROOFING TILE GROUT

I recently had ceramic tile put on our kitchen counter top. It looks very nice but the grout appears to be quite porous and I'm afraid it will stain easily. Is there anything I can apply to make the grout waterproof?

Silicone water repellent, sold for use on leather shoes, will also work on tile grout. Brush it between the tiles with the applicator provided, then wipe any surplus off the tiles before it dries.

REMOVING TILE GROUT

Some of the ceramic tiles on my bathroom wall are chipped and I would like to replace them. I've tried chipping the grout out with a hammer and chisel but this is a very slow job and I'm afraid I'll damage the adjoining tiles. Is there something that will dissolve the grout?

There is no practical solvent that will remove the tile grout, which is basically just white portland cement, but you can make a tool out of an old hacksaw blade that will make it easier to remove the grout. Snap the hacksaw blade in half and use the toothed edge to cut between the tiles. Wrap several layers of masking tape or electrician's tape around the other end to make a handle.

CERAMIC WALL TILES

I am building a bathroom in my basement and would like to apply ceramic tiles to the tub/shower enclosure. Can they be applied directly to the gypsumboard walls?

Yes, but you should not use ordinary gypsumboard, as this can be softened by water absorbed through porous tile grout and cracks in the caulking along the edge of the tub. You should use a special water-resistant gypsumboard, often referred to as "greenboard" because of the surface color used for easy identification. Both the laminated paper face and the gypsum core are water-resistant, designed specifically for the support of tilework in bathrooms and other high-moisture areas. It is installed like other gypsumboard panels except that cut edges and nailheads must be covered with a special sealant, and no joint filler or taping is used in the areas to be tiled. Apply the tiles with a mastic adhesive spread with a notched trowel.

LOOSE TILES ON SHOWER WALL

Our house is only two years old but some of the ceramic tiles around the tub/shower enclosure are coming off the wall. Can you tell me what is causing this and how we can stop it?

A recent study by the National Research Council has found that this is caused by water getting behind the tiles and softening the gypsumboard panelling. If the tiles are coming off just above the tub the problem may be caused by water getting under the bottom of the wall through gaps in the caulking around the tub. Replacing the caulking will correct this.

More often, however, the problem was found to be caused by water seeping through the porous cement grout joints between the tiles. It took less than 10 minutes for water to soak through some of the grouts tested. When the walls were opened for inspection, moisture was found to have soaked right through the gypsumboard, where, on outside walls, it was trapped by the polyethylene vapor barrier. (Tile failure occurs most frequently on outside walls.)

The problem can be prevented by painting the tile grout with a silicone water repellent or white latex paint applied with a small brush. A white latex paste "grout restorer" that is now on the market would probably be even easier to apply. But if the problem has been going on for some time the softened gypsumboard will have to be replaced. If so, be sure to use either a water-resistant gypsumboard generally called "greenboard", or one of the new waterproof cementboards such as Wonderboard or Durock. Also make sure the tile grout is mixed with a latex bonding agent.

TILING OVER WATERPROOF WALLPAPER

Is it possible to apply ceramic tiles over the waterproof wallpaper in my bathroom?

Waterproof wallpaper has a vinyl surface, and nothing sticks to this very well. The wallpaper will be strippable, however. Just peel off the top layer and apply an alkyd primer or an asphalt-based sealer (available where you get the tile) to the exposed backing paper. Then apply the tile adhesive.

CHIMNEYS

CLOSING UNUSED CHIMNEY

We have converted our heating system to electricity, so no longer need the brick chimney. What should we do with it?

There are three things that need to be done: make sure the chimney is structurally safe; keep animals out of it; and seal it to prevent the loss of heated household air and the possiblity of condensation forming inside it.

If the mortar joints have deteriorated and the bricks are crumbling, the chimney should either be repaired or taken down. It will cost less to repair the chimney than to have it demolished and then patch the wall and roof. If the chimney is in good condition, all you need to do is have a sheet metal cap made to fit over the projecting flue tile. The cap should be made of heavy gauge aluminum and held in place with a metal band. For an airtight seal, a bead of caulking compound should be applied to the top of the tile first. If there is no flue tile, the top of the chimney can be covered with a concrete paving slab set in a bed of mortar. The furnace pipe opening in the chimney should also be covered and sealed.

FIREPLACE CHIMNEY FLAKING

The bricks at the top of my fireplace chimney have flaked off very badly in some places, although the house is only 10 years old. What causes this? How can I stop it? And what can I do to repair the damaged bricks?

The flaking or "spalling" is due to water getting into the bricks and then freezing. There are a number of ways this can happen. The chimney may have been capped with porous mortar instead of a solid concrete slab. If a concrete cap was used, it may be cracked, or was not caulked properly around the projecting flue tile. The mortar between the bricks may have deteriorated and needs repointing. Or warm, humid household air may be escaping up the chimney when the fireplace is not being used, causing condensation to form inside it. If the tile lining was not installed properly, the condensation can leak into the bricks. Make sure the fireplace damper is closed after the fire goes out. Tight-fitting glass doors on the fireplace will also help, although neither of these steps will stop air leakage up the chimney completely.

The spalled bricks cannot be repaired, but they can be replaced. Usually the best way to do this is to dismantle the chimney as far as the damage goes and then rebuild it. A less expensive alternative, however, is to reface the chimney with a decorative stucco applied directly to the existing brickwork.

GAS CHIMNEY CRUMBLING

Last summer I noticed pieces of brick from my chimney on the roof. On closer inspection I found that all of the bricks are crumbling and flaking. We converted our heating from oil to gas several years ago. The brick chimney is 25 years old but seems to have a tile lining, which I can see projecting from the top. Can you tell me why this is happening and what I can do to stop it?

Condensation inside the chimney is causing this problem, which is common with old masonry chimneys that have been converted from oil to gas. Gas produces more moisture than oil does when it burns, and it also has a lower flue temperature. Cooler flue gases means that less heat is being wasted up the chimney, of course, but it also causes more condensation.

Your chimney may not have a lining at all. It was common practice 25 or 30 years ago just to put one or two flue tiles at the top. If there is no lining, condensation will seep through the bricks to the outside of the chimney, where the water will freeze and cause the bricks to flake or spall. More serious, however, is the possibility that this can cause the bricks to crumble *inside* the chimney and eventually block the flue, forcing potentially poisonous combustion gases into the house.

Even if you do have flue tiles in the chimney, the mortar joints between them may have deteriorated enough to allow the condensation to leak through into the bricks. In either case, the remedy is to have a Type B metal vent installed inside the masonry chimney. This is now compulsory in many areas when a brick chimney is switched from oil to gas.

INSTALLING A CHIMNEY LINER

I had my furnace converted from oil to gas several years ago. No liner was installed in the brick chimney at that time, but now I understand that it would be a lot safer to have one of these put in. We have a semidetached home, however, and the chimney is located in the common wall between the two units. Is it possible to have a metal liner installed without damaging the house walls?

Yes, either rigid or flexible metal gas liners can be installed with access only to the top and bottom of the chimney.

VENTING DRYER INTO CHIMNEY

We have an unused chimney right beside our basement laundry room. Can this be used as a vent for the clothes dryer?

Because of the high humidity in the dryer exhaust, condensation inside the chimney would be a problem – particularly if it is on an outside wall. It would be much better to put the vent directly through the foundation wall, or even a nearby window.

CONCRETE

CRACKS IN THE BASEMENT FLOOR

My house is about five years old. Two years ago a few small cracks appeared in the basement floor. Now they seem to be getting longer and wider. Does this indicate a serious foundation problem?

No. The basement floor does nothing to support the house. It is just a concrete slab that rests on the ground and is not directly attached to the foundation walls. Even the posts that support the main beam down the centre of the basement do not rest on the floor; they sit on individual concrete footings under the slab. Except for appearances, cracks in the floor are of no consequence unless they leak.

Hairline cracks can be filled with a paint-thick mixture of portland cement powder and water. Larger cracks can be filled with one of the concrete patching materials available at hardware and building supply stores. For best results, water should be brushed on the cracks and allowed to sink in before either of these materials is applied.

REPAIRING OLD FOUNDATION

We have a very old home where the concrete foundation walls are in poor condition, although there is only a little water leakage through them. Some of the concrete has flaked off on the inside near the external ground level, and in a few places the concrete is very soft. I would like to correct these problems so we can finish the basement. Contractors have suggested repairs that vary widely in method and price – from just insulating the walls to adding a new 4 in. block wall on the inside. What should we do?

I do not think there is any inside remedy that would correct all the problems. Loose concrete on the inside can be removed and patched, but the most important step is to dig down to the footings outside, patch any areas where the concrete is soft, then coat the entire wall with a ½ in. layer of cement plaster mixed with an acrylic bonding agent. When this is set it should be covered with a fibrated asphalt foundation coating. Such a treatment should prevent further deterioration of the concrete and allow you to frame, insulate and finish the inside walls without the danger of wood decay from damp concrete.

PATCHING CONCRETE

Some areas of the concrete floor in our garage have flaked off, leaving a number of rough holes. What can I use to fill these and level the floor again?

All hardware and building supply stores carry one or more brands of concrete patching material for jobs like this. While these contain bonding agents that allow them to be applied much thinner than ordinary concrete, the patches will hold much better if you use a chisel to cut the edges of the holes straight down about half and inch. Remove concrete dust, dampen the hole, then brush on a slightly thinned coat of the patching material. While this is still wet fill and level the hole with a patching mixture thick enough to smooth with a trowel.

RESURFACING PATIO

We bought a house with a 10 ft x 16 ft concrete patio slab at the back. The surface of this is badly pitted and one side has sunk about 4 in. (it does not seem to have been bolted to the house properly). Can we apply a new topping to level the slab and provide a new surface? This would vary from 2 in. on one side to about 6 in. on the other.

A slab like this is not supposed to be bolted to the house, but should be sealed to it with a strip of asphalt-impregnated expansion joint material. And the slab should not be perfectly level. A slope of at least ¼ in. to the foot, away from the house is required for surface drainage.

You can apply a new topping as long as it is at least 2 in. thick and is properly mixed and applied, but it is advisable to apply a latex bonding coat to the old slab first. For frost protection, use an air-entrained concrete mix.

SEALING CRACKED CONCRETE

Our concrete steps and front porch are all in one piece, and underneath the porch is a fruit cellar. A large crack has developed from one side of the porch to the other, about a foot back from the top step, and when it rains the water drips into the cold storage room. We have tried several times to fill the crack, but it still leaks. How can we repair it?

Use a cold chisel and hammer to chip out the crack at least and inch deep and ¾ in. wide at the top. Blow out all the dust, then seal the crack at the bottom of the cavity with a flexible caulking compound such as silicone or butyl rubber. Allow this to set for a couple of days, then top the cavity with one of the concrete patching compounds available at hardware and building supply stores.

Chipping out the crack is not an easy job, but it's essential for a waterproof patch.

CONCRETE STEPS FLAKING

I used a de-icing compound on my concrete steps last winter, and after the ice had gone I noticed that the surface of the concrete had flaked away in places. Was this caused by the ice or the de-icing chemical? (It was labelled as Urea Calcium.)

The product you used is a combination of two common de-icing chemicals - urea and calcium chloride. The flaking or spalling is not caused directly by the chemicals, however, but by the increase in the freeze-thaw cycles due to the melting action. Without the de-icer the concrete would have remained below freezing temperature, in other words; with the chemical it thaws and freezes again, causing the concrete to flake or spall. This would not happen if the proper air-entrained concrete had been used. Patch the areas that have flaked, then seal the concrete with a mixture of one part boiled linseed oil and one part kerosene. Let this sink in for an hour or so, then wipe off any surplus with a dry cloth.

CONCRETE PATCHES DON'T MATCH

I had my sidewalk repaired recently, with the result that I now have a number of almost white patches on the grey concrete. Is there some way I can tone these down?

The contractor should have mixed lampblack with the patching material to get a better match. You may be able to make the patches less noticeable by brushing them with a grey latex paint, then wiping most of it off to leave just a slight coloration on the concrete. Mix black universal paint pigment with latex house paint to get the color you need. Test it on some other concrete until you find the right shade.

DOORS

FINISHING A CEDAR DOOR

We recently purchased a solid cedar door with decorative panels for the front of our house. What finish should we put on to retain the natural appearance of the wood?

That depends on what you mean by "natural". If you want to keep the wood the color it is now, you can't do it. Any finish you put on will darken it, and most will add an amber tone. If you don't put anything on the wood, it will weather slowly to a driftwood grey color. The only way to retain the color of fresh-cut cedar is to cover it with a pigmented stain of that color. That looks all right on siding, but it is not very attractive on a front door.

But if you want a clear finish that will show the distinctive grain pattern of the cedar, there are a number of finishes you can use. Thinned linseed oil is often suggested, but this takes a long time to dry, collects dust, and darkens with age. Oil/resin sealers like the Danish oil finishes penetrate deeper and leave the surface texture of the wood virtually unchanged, but they do not provide much physical protection.

Most people prefer a clear film finish such as varnish or urethane. Tests by the National Research Council have shown that the urethanes (or polyurethanes) have a tendency to peel when used outdoors, and that makes them difficult to refinish. The most durable film finish, according to NRC tests, is *four* coats of old-fashioned marine or spar varnish. (This should be applied to all six surfaces of the door - back, front and four edges - to prevent uneven moisture absorption and warping.) Even this finish should be given a new coat every couple of years, before it begins to show deterioration, and it may have to be stripped and re-done about every six years.

GARAGE DOOR CRACKING

My garage door is made of insulated plywood panels. The outside of the bottom panels has become cracked and swollen because of water splashing on the plywood. I plan to replace the plywood on these panels and would like to know what kind to get and what is the best sealer to use?

You must use at least an exterior grade of sanded plywood, but the best type for this job is one with what is called a "medium density overlay". This is a tough, waterproof, plastic-impregnated paper overlay that resists checking and cracking and takes paint very well. You will still have to seal the bottom edge of the plywood panels, however, with several coats of whatever paint you are applying to the face. Sand this edge and fill any lamination gaps before painting.

DOOR MOLDING MELTED

Last spring we added an aluminum storm door to the front of our house, which faces south. During the summer the molding around the four panels on our front door melted and twisted and now look terrible. What has caused this and how can it be corrected?

The glass storm door acts like a greenhouse, trapping the sun's heat in the space between the two doors. Your front door is probably a metal one filled with insulation, and the surface of this can get very hot on a summer day - hot enough to melt plastic molding, anyway. A more expensive type of plastic door molding that will withstand higher temperatures is now available. Contact the door manufacturer and see if he can supply this new molding. The molding panels are attached by means of plugs that snap into holes in the metal door. Pry these off and press the new molding in place, then paint to match the door. If heat-resistant plastic molding is not available, use wood molding fastened with self-tapping metal screws. Countersink the heads and cover with plastic wood.

METAL vs WOOD DOORS

We are considering replacing our front door, but cannot decide between metal and cedar. What are the advantages and disadvantages of both types? Which provides the best insulation?

Metal conducts heat a lot better than wood does, but metal doors are filled with polyurethane foam, which is one of the best insulation materials known. A typical 1 ¾ in. metal door has a total insulation value of about R11; a solid cedar door of the same thickness has an insulation value of about R3.5, and even less if it is panelled. Also, metal doors do not warp, so weatherstripping usually fits much better and there is less air leakage. This is particularly true if you install a pre-hung metal door. On the other hand, metal doors generally cost about 50% more than cedar doors.

The main advantage of a cedar door is its appearance. Most people would agree, I think, that a cedar door with a natural finish looks a lot better than a painted metal door (or a painted cedar door, for that matter). But this has its disadvantages, too; it is very difficult to maintain such a finish on an outside door.

MIRRORED DOORS

Our entrance hall closet has sliding doors with overhead rollers and woodgrain hardboard panels. Can I take these panels out of the metal frame and replace them with mirrors?

Yes, if the doors are no wider than 36 in. and you use mirrored glass 4mm to 6mm thick. As a safety measure, the back of the glass should be covered with peel-off, self adhesive vinyl, as commonly sold for decoration or shelf lining. Also, the sharp edges of the glass should be smoothed with wet carbide abrasive paper or covered with masking tape before it is fitted in the frame.

The correct way to change a panel is to remove the door, push out the roller hangers and bottom guides, then take off the frame sections. Measure the panel to get the exact size of the mirror and have it delivered to your house. Reassemble the frame on the mirror (after treating it as described above), snap the hangers and bottom guides in place, then rehang.

But glass is a tricky material to handle in large sheets, and I don't really recommend this as a do-it-yourself job. If the doors are wider than 36 in., you'll need a new heavy-duty frame with top and bottom rollers, anyway. Better give the job to an expert and let him worry about breaking the glass or scratching the mirrors.

REPAINTING A METAL DOOR

When the paint on our metal front door began to peel last year I scraped it down to bare metal and repainted it with two coats of a premium "rustproof" paint. The job was done during hot weather and I left about two days of drying time between coats. Now it is peeling again. What did I do wrong?

The metal was probably too hot when you painted it. This causes the solvent to evaporate so quickly that the film-forming polymers in the paint do not have time to form a bond with the metal. The door should have been allowed to cool in the shade for an hour or two before the paint was applied.

It would also help to use a primer on the bare metal before painting. I know that not all "rustproof" paints require this, but some do and others admit that it might help. Virtually all metal doors are made of preprimed galvanized steel, but you will have removed the primer when you scraped the original paint off. Before you repaint, apply a primer labelled as being for use on *galvanized* metal. Then apply two coats of an alkyd enamel or, if you prefer, one of the "rustproof" paints.

PATIO DOOR STICKING

Our aluminum patio door does not slide smoothly any more. It is still in its track but is very hard to move. Is there any way I can fix this?

The problem could be caused by the door riding too high in the bottom track causing it to stick in the top track. (This could also be due to the beam over the doorway having sagged slightly.) The remedy for this is to lower the door by adjusting the bottom rollers. This can be done by turning a screw that is hidden in a hole at the bottom edge of the sliding door, one on each side for the two rollers. It is not necessary to remove the door to do this.

But sometimes the problem is caused by nothing more than dirt or some other obstruction blocking the bottom rollers. To get at this you have to remove the door. Lower the door as far as it will go by adjusting the height of the rollers as described above, then lift the door up into the top track so you can pull it cut at the bottom – a 2-man job but otherwise fairly easy. Examine and clean the rollers. They do not need to be lubricated.

Too often, however, you will find that the problem is a broken wheel. To fix this it is usually necessary to remove the bottom rail from the door, take out the broken roller and get a replacement from the door manufacturer or a firm that handles parts and service. You may be able to get the name of such a company from your hardware or building supply store, or you can look in the Yellow Pages under Doors - Rolling & Sliding.

RAISING A POCKET DOOR

We recently had a thick carpet installed, and now our pocket door catches on this when we slide it open. How can we raise the door?

You can't, but you can cut enough off the bottom to clear the carpet. You'll have to remove the door to do this. A pocket door must be swung out sideways at the bottom so the rollers can be lifted off the overhead trick, the same way that sliding wardrobe doors are removed. But to do this you must first remove the jamb and casing from the pocket side of the doorway in order to provide enough clearance to swing the door out.

TRIMMING A PLYWOOD DOOR

We had deep pile carpeting and a thick underpad laid throughout our house recently, and now most of the interior doors are rubbing on the carpet. How can we shorten the hollow plywood doors?

There should be at least an inch and a half of solid wood at the bottom of the doors, and this will let you saw off enough to provide adequate clearance over the carpet. Remove the hinge pins and lay the door on a pair of sawhorses. Measure the amount to be trimmed, then use a metal straightedge and a razor knife to score the plywood. Do this on both sides of the door. Saw on the lower side of this cut to prevent the edges of the plywood from chipping. Sandpaper the bottom of the door before rehanging.

SOLID DOOR WARPS IN WINTER

Our front door has a solid wood core with mahogany veneer. Every winter it warps inwards at the top and bottom on the latch side. When summer comes, it's flat again. How can we keep this from happening?

This summer, take the door off its hinges and apply three or four coats of satin urethane varnish to the inside face of the door and all four edges. This should prevent differences in the moisture content of the inside and outside wood surfaces that cause the door to warp.

DRIVEWAYS

DRIVEWAY SEALER TRACKS INTO HOUSE

I painted my asphalt driveway with a coal tar sealer that has tracked into the house, leaving yellowish stains on the steps, carpet and white vinyl floor. How can I remove these and what can I do to prevent any more?

The only solvent that works on coal tar is toluene, which happens to be one of the main ingredients of lacquer thinner, so you can use this to remove tar stains from most materials. You'll find it doesn't work too well on white vinyl, however, because the stain tends to penetrate into the plastic.

If you applied the driveway sealer early in the year, cold weather may have kept it from drying properly. Coal tar emulsion should not be walked on for 24 hours, even in hot weather. Putting it on too thick will also make it dry slowly, and may keep the undersurface tacky for weeks. Two thin layers are much better than one thick one.

The tar also will not dry properly if the driveway gets wet before the sealer dries; even a light drizzle will do it. Applying the sealer over oily patches on the driveway can also produce sticky spots. Such areas should be cleaned off first with a degreasing compound or trisodium phosphate (wet the spot, sprinkle with TSP crystals, brush in, leave 15 minutes, brush again, then hose off).

If your driveway hasn't dried properly by the time you read this, the best remedy is to apply a special acrylic sealer/hardener - Universal Tar Hardener, made by Universal Coatings Company, 58 Hymus Road, Scarborough, Ontario M1L 2C7.

LAYING A CONCRETE DRIVEWAY

We want to have our dirt driveway paved with concrete, but are getting many different opinions on how this should be done. Some people suggest putting down several inches of gravel first. Others say to use limestone or plastic film. One contractor insists on using steel reinforcing mesh in the concrete. The recommended thickness has varied from 2 to 6 in. We have also heard stories about salt damage and would like to know how to prevent this.

Details will vary to some extent depending on site conditions, of course, but according to the Canadian Portland Cement Association, here are the basic requirements for a good concrete driveway (or any slab on grade).

The best base is firm, undisturbed earth, simply cut back and levelled at the required depth. Shallow depressions can be filled with tamped earth. Granular fill such as gravel, crushed rock or limestone screenings is only required if the present earth level is too low. Passenger cars need a driveway slab no more than 4 in. (100mm) thick. If light trucks are expected, it should be 5 in. (125mm) thick. Steel reinforcing mesh serves no useful purpose in a ground-supported slab, and is not recommended by the CPCA.

The concrete mix should be specified at a strength of 30MPa (megapascals) with 6% to 8% air entrainment to prevent frost damage. Where the driveway will meet the garage floor, house foundation, sidewalk, or other solid construction, the two surfaces should be separated by an "isolation joint", usually a strip of asphalt-impregnated fibreboard. Other than poor concrete, the most common cause of surface failure is attempting to finish the concrete too soon, before the surface water has evaporated and the concrete is firm enough to be stepped on without making an impression more than a quarter of an inch deep. (This usually takes about an hour but can be twice as long if the temperature is low.) Overworking the fresh concrete can make the surface soft and powdery, causing it to wear away in a year or two and expose the rough aggregate. It is also the cause of flaking or scaling. (Contrary to popular opinion, these problems are NOT caused by road salt, which has little or no effect on good concrete that was properly finished.)

Only when the concrete has started to firm up (as described above) can the surface be given a final levelling by hand with a wood or metal float. A powerdriven float or trowel should NOT be used. At this stage, too, one-inch-deep "control joints" should be cut in the concrete. These are required every 10 ft., in both width and length, to prevent unsightly random cracks in the concrete due to shrinkage as it hardens and cures. Control joints will confine the cracks to these precut groves, where they cannot be seen. A single driveway should have crosswise control joints every 10 ft. A double driveway also requires a control joint down the centre, dividing the concrete into 10-ft-square sections, more or less.

At the same time as the control joints are being cut, the surface of the driveway should be brushed with a stiff broom to give a non-skid finish.

The final requirement, and a very important one, is to keep the concrete *continuously* wet for a period of at least five days in warm weather and seven days in cool weather so it will harden properly. The driveway can be wet with a hose and then covered with polyethylene film or waterproof paper; or a special curing compound can be sprayed on the concrete as soon as it is finished (no wetting is necessary with this method, and the coating will eventually wear off).

SEALING A BRICK DRIVEWAY

Our driveway is surfaced with interlocking paving bricks that look great except for a large oil stain left by a friend's car. How can I get rid of this, and what can I do to protect the driveway from similar stains?

First use one of the grease removers sold at hardware and auto supply stores. Products such as Gunk, Dunk, Polyclens and Motomaster Engine Cleaner will emulsify the oil so it can be removed with a brush and hose. If a deeper stain remains, use the "poultice" treatment. Add petroleum solvent (Varsol, etc.) to powdered white chalk to make a paste that can be spread on the stain area about a quarter of an inch thick. Cover with polyethylene film or plastic food wrap taped down around the edges. Leave this for an hour or so, remove the plastic and allow the chalk to dry thoroughly, then brush off. If you're lucky, the oil stain will go with it. Repeat if necessary.

To prevent such stains, apply one of the clear acrylic masonry sealers available from building supply stores and companies that sell or install interlocking paving stones. Two sealers that leave no discernible finish are Hydrozo and Thompson's 101 Water Seal. Three brands that give the paving a wet look and darken the color are Thoroglaze, Watco Tile & Brick Sealer and Benjamin Moore's Silicone Acrylic Concrete Stain (clear). Apply as directed by the manufacturer.

WEEDS GROWING THROUGH DRIVEWAY

What chemical can I use to kill weeds and grass growing through our asphalt driveway?

Any general herbicide can be used. Ordinary table salt also works well. So does boiling water.

ELECTRICITY

COST OF USING HEATING CABLE

We used an electric heating cable on our roof this winter to prevent ice dams from forming. How can we figure out how much this cost to operate?

That depends on the length of the cable and the time it was on. This type of cable is generally rated at five watts per foot – a 50 ft (15m) cable uses as much electricity as a 250-watt light bulb, in other words. If you left it on all day it would use 6000 watt-hours, or six kilowatt-hours, which will cost you around 25 to 30 cents, depending on the rate in your area. That would be $7.50 to $9 a month if you left the cable on all the time. (If you have more or less cable than the 50 ft I have used as an example

here, adjust these figures accordingly.) But a roof de-icing cable should not be turned on, or plugged in, unless there is snow on the roof and some sign of ice forming along the eavestrough edge. Any other time you are only wasting electricity.

DO DIMMERS SAVE ELECTRICITY?

We have dimmer switches on our living room lights. Do they really reduce the amount of electricity used, or is it just dissipated somewhere else?

At one time, dimmers were variable transformers that reduced the voltage delivered to the light. These were not only bulky and expensive but also wasted some of the electricity in the form of heat. The heart of a modern dimmer is a tiny silicon diode that cuts off the pulses of alternating current before they reach their peak voltage. It produces very little heat. And since you only pay for the electricity that is used, it does reduce your hydro bills.

DO-IT-YOURSELF WIRING vs INSURANCE

It is obvious from the large display of electric wiring supplies in every hardware store that a lot of homeowners do this work themselves, and I would be willing to bet that very few of them obtain a permit or have the work inspected. I have done such wiring myself, but must add that I have taken the trouble to learn how it should be done, and do it very carefully, with great respect for the hazards of electricity. My question is this: Does such work nullify insurance coverage on the house? I have been told that it does.

This is a tricky question, but a very good one, and I have discussed it with a number of claims experts in the insurance business. It is tricky because there is no set, written industry-wide policy on this question. Every company makes its own decisions, and each claim must be looked at separately.

Nevertheless, the general attitude to this question does seem to be quite consistent, and it is this: The insurance on your house covers specified perils, such as fire, and there is no exclusion for accidental damage that you may have caused yourself. You (or anyone in your immediate family) may have spilled some gasoline in the basement, set the curtains on fire with a propane torch, or installed a light fixture incorrectly (and illegally). As long as the damage was unintentional the insurance coverage remains in force - ignorance, carelessness or stupidity notwithstanding.

But if the damage was caused by faulty work done by an outsider – a workman, a relative, a friend – the insurance company does have the right to sue them, in your name, for recovery of the damages. So doing the wiring on your own home will not cancel your insurance, but if a friend asks you to help him do some wiring in *his* house, think twice about it.

Nevertheless, there are good reasons for obtaining a permit and having the work inspected. Building regulations require it, for one thing, and family safety is certainly another.

ELECTRIC HEAT REQUIREMENTS

We are going to convert an attached garage to a family room. The walls and ceiling will be insulated. How can we determine the size of electric baseboard heaters this room will require?

For a rough estimate, you can figure on 10 watts per square foot of floor area, but the actual requirement may be half or twice that, depending on the temperature in your area and the amount of insulation you have. The only accurate way to determine the heating requirement is by making a heat loss calculation. Your electric utility will do this for you, and also determine whether your present service capacity can take the extra load.

EXTENDING SWITCH BOXES

I am putting cedar V-joint panelling on my bathroom walls. How do I move the electrical outlet boxes so they will be flush with the new panelling and provide a fireproof enclosure for the switches and duplex outlets - without having to tear the walls apart?

There is a simple remedy. Metal sections are available that fit over the end of the wiring box. They are called switch box extensions, or SBEX, are adjustable up to ⅞ in., and can be purchased at any electrical supply store.

FLICKERING LIGHTS

Certain lights in our house come on OK, then begin to flicker and go off all at once. Other lights and outlets in the house are unaffected. We had an electrician check the connections in the fuse panel and the service meter, but he said he couldn't find anything wrong.

The electrician should have checked the wiring in the circuit where the problem is located. There must be a loose connection there some-

where. The first thing to do is find out which outlets and light fixtures are on this circuit. You can do this by removing the fuse that controls this circuit and then testing *every light and outlet inside and outside the house.* (Use a light bulb on a short extension cord to check the plug-in outlets.) All the ones that have no power are on this faulty circuit.

The next time the lights go off, check to see if all the lights and outlets in this circuit are off. I think you will find that at least one still has power. This will show that the circuit is receiving power from the service panel, and that the loose connection is not far from the live outlet. If there is an outdoor outlet in the circuit, this is the most likely location of the problem.

Unless you have had experience working with electric wiring, leave the repair work to a licensed electrician - preferably not the one who checked the panel. I strongly recommend that you leave the fuse out of that circuit until you get it fixed.

FLUORESCENT FIXTURE WON'T WORK

I bought a 4 ft, 2-tube fluorescent light fixture for my basement workshop and connected it to a duplex outlet with lamp cord and a 2-prong plug. The light doesn't always come on when I plug it in. What's wrong?

Failure of the fluorescent fixture to light could be due to a loose connection, of course, but more likely it's caused by the lack of ground wire connected to the metal fixture box.

A mounted fixture like this is not supposed to be wired with lamp cord, in any case. It should be wired into an available house circuit through a wall switch, using standard 14-gauge, 2-wire cable (which actually contains three wires, counting the bare ground wire). The ground wire is connected to the metal housing of the fluorescent fixture and to the electrical outlet box. It is required not only for safety, to prevent you getting a shock if there is a short circuit in the fixture, but also for the proper operation of the fluorescent ballast and starter circuit.

FREE LIGHT?

Our house is heated by electricity. A friend tells us we can burn as many lights in the house as we want to all winter without it costing us anything. That can't be true, can it?

Yes it can. Electricity produces the same amount of heat whether you use it in a toaster, electric furnace, baseboard heater or lighting. Even the light is converted to heat when it hits a wall, floor, ceiling or anything else in the room. So electricity consumed by your lights will reduce, by the same amount, the electricity used by the heating system. In a sense, then, the light is free. This only works in winter, however.

GROUNDING AN OUTDOOR OUTLET

I have an old house with electric wiring that is not grounded. The only outlet I'm worried about is an outside one that I use for the power mower, sometimes when the grass is wet. Is there any way I can ground this outlet to protect myself?

The best way to do it is to ask an electrician to run a ground wire from the outlet box back to the main service panel. But if you want to do the job yourself, simply run a length of #12 copper wire from the green ground screw on the duplex receptacle to a cold water pipe inside the house. Use a metal grounding strap to make the connection to the pipe.

Even with a ground outlet, however, you can still receive a dangerous shock if the ground is wet and there is a small amount of current leakage - too small to blow a fuse - in the appliance you are touching. Because of this, the Canadian Electrical Code now requires a special type of duplex receptacle in outdoor outlets. This contains a device that senses the current leakage and opens the circuit fast enough to prevent any injury. It is called a ground fault circuit interrupter (GFCI) receptacle, and is easy to install.

LIGHT BULB BRIGHTENS

When our refrigerator starts up, the ceiling light in our kitchen brightens. This bulb keeps burning out, too, and has to be replaced every few weeks, it seems. What could be causing this?

A poor ground connection in the neutral (white) wiring can cause a voltage increase in one circuit when power is drawn from another. The most likely place for the poor connection is back at the main service panel. You'd better ask an electrician to look at this.

ADJUSTING WATER TEMPERATURE

I had my gas water heater replaced with an electric one. The temperature control on the old one was on the outside of the tank and we had adjusted it to a suitable temperature. The adjustments on the new electric tank must be done by an electrician, I was told. I asked the installer what temperature the new tank was set for and he replied: "Normal, 150°". I don't think this can be normal at all. We find it much too hot, and I'm sure it's dangerous for adults as well as children. What is the proper setting?

Medical and safety authorities agree that water at 150° F (65°C) is indeed hazardous, particularly for children and seniors, although that was the standard setting for many years. CSA standards now require that electric water heaters be set at 140°F (60°C) and carry a warning label about higher temperatures. There are still a lot of water heaters around that were manufactured before these standards came into force, but the installer should adjust the thermostat to the new setting and apply the warning label.

Some authorities believe that the temperature should be even lower - 120°F (49°C) is often recommended - but other experts point out that most animal fats melt at 128°F (47°C), and that the tank temperature needs to be a little higher than that to allow for heat loss in the pipes. Also, automatic dishwashers require a water temperature of 140°F. This seems like the most practical setting for the heater, but water at this temperature must still be used with caution and common sense.

You can adjust the temperature setting yourself very easily. First disconnect the fuse, circuit breaker or switch that controls the water heater (it should be marked on the service panel). Most electric hot water tanks have two heating elements, each with its own thermostat. These are located behind access panels near the top and bottom of the tank. Remove the panels, push the insulation aside, if necessary, and use a screwdriver to adjust the temperature setting on the thermostat dials. Both thermostats should have the same setting. Do not move any other screws or wires.

FIREPLACES

GLASS DOORS ON FIREPLACE

Our fireplace puts out a lot of heat, but we are told it would work much better if we added glass doors. Can you tell us if this would improve its performance?

There are two different factors involved here. One is the amount of heat given off by the fireplace; the other is its heating efficiency - the difference between the amount of heat the fireplace radiates into the room, and the amount of cold air it draws in to maintain the chimney draft. Because all of the air that goes up the chimney must be replaced by cold outside air drawn into the house, most open fireplaces probably operate at a net heat loss during cold weather. They are comforting and interesting to look at, but do nothing to reduce your heating bills. (No one expects a TV set to pay for itself, however.)

Adding glass doors increases the efficiency of a fireplace because not as much air is drawn up the chimney. But glass doors also reduce very severely the amount of heat that is radiated into the room. Opening the glass doors will overcome that, of course, but lowers the efficiency again. It also eliminates the protection glass doors provide against fire damage from flying sparks or hot coals.

Another advantage of glass doors is that they allow you to close the fire down completely at bedtime and prevent heat loss up the chimney during the night.

Because glass doors increase the temperature inside the firebox, they cannot be used with most metal fireplaces. If you have one of these, check with the manufacturer to see if it is approved for use with glass doors.

You must also be careful not to build too large a fire or allow burning wood to touch the glass. Make sure, too, that the doors are made of tempered glass; this can still break with excessive heat, but it crumbles instead of shattering as ordinary glass will do. A number of such cases have been reported. As a further protection against this hazard, many stores specializing in fireplace equipment will not install glass doors on a fireplace that is less than 15 in. deep.

CLEANING GLASS FIREPLACE DOORS

We bought a set of glass doors for our fireplace to improve its efficiency. They work very well, but the glass gets discolored by a deposit of some kind that won't come off with ordinary window cleaners. What should I use?

Oven cleaner will usually remove it, but you can also use one of the liquid drain cleaners. These strong caustic solutions must be handled very carefully, however. Keep them off everything but the glass.

COLD DRAFT FROM GAS FIREPLACE

We installed a gas fireplace last winter and had trouble with the cold air that came down the vent pipe when the fireplace was not being used. As a result, the temperature in our living room was 5°C lower than the rest of the house most of the time. We would like to put a damper of some kind in the vent pipe so we can shut this when the fireplace is not being used.

Safety regulations forbid the use of a manual damper in a gas fireplace. The vent must be left open at all times, *even when the fireplace is not being used.*

CLEANING STONE FIREPLACE

I forgot to open the damper before I started a fire in our fieldstone fireplace. How can I remove the smoke stain?

Oven cleaner will do it. So will a solution of one heaping tablespoon of trisodium phosphate (TSP) to a quart of water.

CREOSOTE SMELL FROM FIREPLACE

Although our fireplace is clean and rarely used now, we still get an odor from it like wet ashes or creosote every once in a while. How can we stop this?

The odor is caused by downdrafts that leak past the fireplace damper; these never fit very tightly. You can stop the downdraft by having a tight-fitting plywood plug made for the fireplace opening (this can be covered with fabric or other decorative material), or by installing a type of fireplace damper that fits on top of the chimney. The latter is available from stores that specialize in fireplaces and wood stoves.

FIREPLACE TURNS FURNACE ON

We have a new home with a strange problem. Whenever we light the fireplace in the main floor family room the furnace comes on and stays on as long as the fireplace is burning. We have to switch the furnace off entirely to keep the house from getting too hot. Neither the builder nor the furnace serviceman can find anything wrong.

Only the thermostat can turn the furnace on, so cool air must be blowing on it somehow when the fireplace is burning. Actually, there is a very simple explanation. A fireplace draws a lot of air out of the house, creating a slight vacuum that pulls in replacement air through doors, windows and other leakage points. Perhaps the thermostat is close enough to one of these to be affected by the draft. If no such source can be located, the cool air may be coming through the hole in the wall behind the thermostat itself, where the control wires run to the furnace. This hole should be sealed with caulking compound, but seldom is. Remove the thermostat from the wall and plug the wire hole.

INSTALLING A GAS FIREPLACE

I am building a family room in my basement and would like to put a gas fireplace in it, but I do not want to have to put a vent up through two floors and the roof. We already have an insulated metal vent for our gas furnace and water heater. Can a gas fireplace be connected to this?

According to the national installation code for gas appliances, a self-contained gas fireplace unit can be connected to an existing furnace vent as long as certain conditions are met. Factors that must be considered are the size and height of the vent, the distance the fireplace will be from it, and the total heat output (or gas consumption) of the appliances that are connected to it. Local codes may have other restrictions. In most cases, however, a separate vent will be required for a gas fireplace. This can be installed on the outside of the house to avoid having to cut through floors and ceilings. Firms that sell and install these units will be able to give you more information about their venting requirements.

CLOSING A GAS FIREPLACE

I am concerned about the heat that is being lost during cold weather from our old gas-fired fireplace, which is seldom used. I can't find a damper of any kind in the chimney. Should I have one installed?

Safety regulations prohibit manually-controlled dampers in gas-fired appliance vents, but there is no reason why you can't put a plywood plug in the fireplace opening. You can use weatherstripping around the edge to get a tight seal, and the front can be covered with a decorative fabric or wallpaper.

METAL FIREPLACE HAS BUCKLED

The back panel of my sheet metal fireplace has buckled very badly. What would cause this? Is it dangerous?

Some distortion of the metal is normal and no cause for concern unless one of the seams opens up, in which case the fireplace should be replaced. The problem is caused by heat, of course, and is usually due to having fires that are too hot. The use of man-made firelogs (the wax-and-sawdust-type) in sheet metal fireplaces is discouraged for this reason; when these logs break apart while they are burning, the fire can get hot enough to warp the sheet metal.

Excessive temperature can also be caused by overloading the fireplace in an attempt to heat the entire house with it. Safety authorities point out that these so-called "zero clearance" sheet metal fireplaces should only be used for supplementary heating. They are not made to burn constantly with a full fuel load.

FIREPLACE MORTAR CRUMBLING

The mortar between the bricks inside our fireplace is crumbling very badly. In some places I can stick the tip of my finger in a half an inch or more. Our house is only six years old but we have used the fireplace regularly. Is the mortar problem dangerous?

I don't think it is dangerous yet, but it could be if it is not repaired. From your description it appears that common mortar (and perhaps common brick, too) was used in the firebox. The building code requires the firebox to be lined with heat-resistant firebrick laid with a high-temperature "refractory" mortar, which is usually no more than 1/8 in. thick. I suggest that you scrape out all the loose mortar and replace it with a premixed refractory mortar. This is available from building supply stores and brick companies.

PLASTER BULGING OVER FIREPLACE

We have lived in our house ever since it was built 30 years ago, and have never used the fireplace. In the past few years we have noticed a discoloration on the plaster wall above the fireplace, and recently it has begun to bulge out in one area. We checked the attic and it is perfectly dry. We also had the flashing around the chimney checked and repaired by a roofer. What do you think is the trouble?

I suspect that you don't have a tile flue lining in the old chimney, and this is allowing rainwater to seep through the bricks and mortar into the plaster wall. (You can check the lining by looking up the chimney with a mirror on a bright day.)

The best remedy is to put a raincap on the top of the chimney. You can seal it completely if you don't plan to use the fireplace, and this will also prevent the loss of warm air up the chimney during the winter.

To repair the wall you have to remove all the loose plaster and fill the hole with plaster of paris or other powder patching material that is mixed with water. Fill the hole about two-thirds full on the first application. Let this dry thoroughly, then fill it level and smooth with a large trowel. When dry, sand lightly and apply a third coat to compensate for the shrinkage. A very thin fourth coat may be necessary to achieve an invisible patch.

POLISHING A SLATE HEARTH

We had a brick fireplace and raised slate hearth installed in our basement family room a few months ago. When the workman finished he wiped the slate with lemon oil. This looked black and shiny for a while but I was afraid to sit on it or put anything on it because of the oil. After a few weeks the shine was gone and the slate turned grey. What is the best way to put a shine on slate?

So-called "lemon oil" is really just a volatile petroleum distillate scented with a few drops of lemon essence. This evaporates quite quickly, and has left the slate in its natural grey color. If you don't like this you can darken the color and give it a glossy finish with a water-based floor wax or a clear acrylic polish. Both of these are widely sold for use on vinyl flooring. This finish will also prevent food spills from staining the slate.

FLOORS

REINFORCING BOUNCY FLOOR

Our house is only 10 years old, but the floor is so bouncy it's positively uncomfortable to walk on, and I get the impression it's not strong enough to support a crowd. Is there any way I can correct this? The basement is unfinished, so I can reach the floor from underneath without any trouble.

The best remedy for this problem is to double several of the floor joists. You will have to remove the 2x2 bridging between the joists in order to place the reinforcing joists beside them. These should be the same dimension as the existing joists (eg: 2x8) but only long enough to span the distance from the main beam to the foundation wall. Fasten the new joists to the existing one with three rows of 3 in. common nails stagger-spaced about 10 in. apart the full length of the joist. Nail 13 in. lengths of 2x4 between the joists in place of the bridging that was removed.

CIGARETTE BURN ON VINYL FLOOR

I dropped a lighted cigarette on my new cushion vinyl floor in the kitchen and it left a deep burn about one centimeter in diameter. Is there anything I can patch this with?

If the floor is white or off-white you can fill the burn with a 2-part epoxy plumber's paste. It would be difficult to match a color with this material, however. A better remedy in this case is to cut out the burn and replace it with a patch of the same material, which can be taken from under the fridge if you don't have any scraps of the flooring left. Hobby shops specializing in leathercraft supplies sell circular cutters in various sizes. Get one a little larger than the burn and also use it to cut a matching patch. A dab of carpenter's glue or resin adhesive will hold the patch in place, or you can weld the edges with a vinyl adhesive.

REMOVING CORK TILES

I have a cork wall with some damaged tiles. How can I remove these so they can be replaced? They are the peel-off, self-stick type, and they are stuck very firmly.

A putty knife is the best tool to use. To avoid damaging the adjoining tiles, make a straight cut in the center of the damaged tile and insert the putty knife there, then work out to the edges.

RESTORING A CORK FLOOR

We have had a cork tile floor in our living area since 1958, and it has worn beautifully - or more correctly, it has hardly worn at all. It does look a bit grungy in spots, however, probably because of wax buildup and dirt, and we would like to know how to restore it to its original appearance.

Cork is simply a form of wood, of course, and its treatment as flooring is much the same as you would give a wood floor. The wax and dirt buildup can be removed with a wax stripper labelled as being suitable for use on wood floors. This may be all the restoration work the cork floor needs, but if marks remain, give the floor a light sanding with #80 paper and a light-weight orbital or belt sander, preferably one with a vacuum attachment. Do not use a heavy sander meant for hardwood floors; this will cut through the soft cork too quickly. The sanded cork tiles can be left natural, rubbed with paste wax and buffed, or given two coats of urethane floor varnish, sanding lightly between coats.

CARE OF MARBLE FLOOR

We recently purchased a 25-year-old home that has a marble floor in the entrance hall. The shade varies from white to pale salmon but it has been discolored by a wax buildup, particularly around the edges. How can I remove this without harming the marble, and what should I put on afterwards to protect the surface?

Paste wax should not be used on marble floors. If that's what you have, it can be removed with petroleum solvent (Varsol, Shelsol) and some clean cloths. The proper sealer-polish for marble is a clear acrylic liquid polish, as sold for use on resilient floors. Terrazzo/slate sealers can also be used on marble. Both of these can build up and discolor the marble in time, too, but can be removed with a strong ammonia solution (half a cup to a quart of water) or one of the commercial wax strippers.

FINISHING OAK FLOORS

We have an older home with oak floors that are badly in need of refinishing. We are going to have the work done by professionals, but first we must decide what finish we want. Some people say that urethane is best, but we find this too glossy. Is there a natural-looking wood finish that can be used on an oak floor? We also think it might be nice to darken the wood with a stain. Is this practical? Please tell us how the work should be done so we can make sure we get what we want.

Urethane is the toughest floor finish, but it doesn't have to be glossy; satin urethane is also available, and it requires less attention because traffic wear is less apparent. The proper procedure for refinishing the floor is to sand it down to bare wood, starting with #40 paper and

ending with #80, then dust or vacuum thoroughly. A walnut stain looks very good on oak, and the darker color does not show dirt or or scuff marks as easily. But when a stain is to be applied, sand the floor with a finer paper, such as #120. Also make sure the stain is compatable with urethane; some contain metallic stearates or soaps that this finish does not adhere to very well.

At least two coats of urethane finish should be applied. Some manufacturers recommend thinning the first coat slightly; others do not. Professional floor finishers often substitute a fast-drying lacquer for the first coat in order to save time, but none of the urethane manufacturers recommend this.

It is also important not to let the first coat of urethane dry too hard before the next is applied. Twenty-four hours is generally considered the maximum time to allow between coats. If it dries much longer than that, it should be sanded lightly before the next coat is applied.

The easiest finish to apply and maintain is a penetrating oil/resin sealer such as one of the Danish oil finishes. These are available with built-in stains, if desired. The floor should be given a final sanding with #120 paper or #0000 steel wool before the sealer is applied. The finish is simply brushed on, allowed to sink in for 15 minutes or so, *then wiped off.* (It is very important to remove all surplus finish at this time.) After 24 hours the floor should be buffed with fine steel wool and then vacuumed before a second coat of sealer is applied the same way as the first. Buff again with fine steel wool when dry and then apply a good paste wax and buff with an electric polisher.

One advantage of a penetrating finish like this is that it provides a soft, satin sheen that can be touched up at any time simply by sanding the worn or damaged area and applying another coat of finish.

OAK FLOOR OVER CONCRETE

I have bought an apartment in a high-rise condominium that is still being built. The floors are concrete and I would like to have oak plank flooring put down instead of carpeting. Can this be done?

Solid oak *parquet* tile flooring can be applied directly to concrete with adhesive, but solid oak plank or strip flooring should be nailed to a plywood underlay that is glued in place. There is also a laminated, prefinished plank flooring (not solid oak) that is flexible enough to be glued directly to concrete. Discuss these with the builder.

CARE OF PARQUET FLOOR

We have bought an older house with parquet floors that need cleaning and polishing. How should we go about it?

Any polish buildup should be taken off with a solvent-type wax remover made for use on hardwood floors. Do the floor in sections, about 4 square feet at a time. Apply the remover to one section, let it stand for a few minutes, then apply it to the next section and let it stay there while you scrub the softened wax off the first section with a nylon scouring pad or steel wool. Continue to leapfrog in this way until the entire floor has been cleaned.

For a final surface cleaning, go over the floor with fine steel wool pads on an electric floor polisher, then apply a paste or liquid *solvent-based* wax. Polish as directed. From then on, the floor need only be dusted regularly, cleaned with a *damp* cloth or sponge when necessary, and waxed once or twice a year.

REFINISHING A PARQUET FLOOR

We have run into a problem trying to apply a urethane finish to our oak parquet tile floor. The factory finish on the tiles got dull very quickly, so we carefully removed the wax we had put on them and then applied two coats of a well-known brand of urethane floor finish. The floor looked great at first, but in less than a year the new finish began to peel off. Now, some months later, the urethane can be lifted off in strips with a putty knife. What did we do wrong?

The proper way to refinish any hardwood floor is to sand off the old finish and start fresh. This is particularly important when using urethane, which is notoriously incompatable with other finishes - and even with itself if the previous coat has dried very hard.

The remedy is to have the floor sanded down to bare wood, then refinished with two coats of satin or gloss urethane. (A lacquer sealer should NOT be used.) If you want to do the job yourself, you can rent a commercial floor sander and use it as directed, finishing with #100 or #120 paper. You'll also need a small belt sander for the edges and corners. Vacuum thoroughly before applying the finish, and follow the directions on the label very carefully.

SPOTS ON PARQUET FLOOR

We had parquet floor tiles laid directly on the concrete in our basement a few years ago. Last summer they developed black spots that look as if moisture is coming up underneath them, although the concrete was poured on 6 in. of crushed stone, was always perfectly dry, and was given a coat of sealer before the tiles were laid. The spots are almost black.

These sound like water stains, and they are most likely caused by condensation forming on the cold floor during humid summer weather. Such stains can be removed by applying a concentrated solution of oxalic acid crystals. These can be obtained from any drug store; they may even have them as the shelves labelled as Rust Remover (the label will say "contains oxalic acid"). ZUD Rust Remover, sold at supermarkets, will also do the job.

Dissolve a teaspoon in half a cup of warm water, then soak a piece of cloth in this solution and place it on the stain, which should be bleached out within 20 minutes or so. Rinse with plain water.

The way to prevent this trouble recurring is to use a dehumidifier in the basement during humid weather.

QUARRY TILE OVER VINYL

I would like to put down a quarry tile floor in my kitchen. It presently consists of vinyl tile on ¾ in. plywood, and the kitchen floor joists are exposed in the basement. Do I need to reinforce the floor before laying ceramic tile? How do I remove the vinyl tile? What kind of mortar should I use?

Unless the kitchen floor is unusually springy there should be no need to reinforce it. And if the present tile is firmly attached, there is no need to remove it.

Clean the floor thoroughly with a commercial wax remover or a solution of 1 cup of liquid ammonia and ¼ cup of powdered floor cleaner to 2 quarts of water. Apply the quarry tile with mastic adhesive sold for this purpose, using a notched trowel. Use a premixed, precolored grout.

CARE OF QUARRY TILE FLOOR

We had a quarry tile floor put down in our hallway. I cleaned it first with muriatic acid and water and then put on two coats of silicone and three coats of a product that was

supposed to seal the surface. But spots keep appearing on it and my attempts to touch them up with paste wax have not been successful. Any advice you can give me would be much appreciated.

Plain, unglazed quarry tile is a very attractive, durable flooring material that is easy to maintain, and most tile experts agree that it should be left alone. Homeowners' attempts to improve it with silicones, acrylics, waxes and assorted sealers too often lead to the type of problem you are having. I have no idea which one is causing the spots, but my advice is to remove them all and get back to the plain quarry tile. The wax and the three coats of sealer can be removed with a wax stripper sold for use on vinyl floors. Petroleum solvent or paint thinner will take off most of the silicone.

REMOVING WAX FROM TERRAZZO

How can I remove a heavy wax buildup from a terrazzo floor? I have tried wax remover, hot water and vinegar, several household cleaners and a lot of hard scrubbing, but none of them worked. How can I restore color and shine to the floor?

Floor polish manufacturers use the word "wax" very loosely. It is often used for products that are not waxes at all, but water solutions of acrylic polymers that produce a clear, glossy, protective film that is similar to a lacquer or varnish. Unlike these finishes, however, the acrylic polishes can be removed very easily, using a solution of 1 cup of liquid ammonia, 1/4 cup of powdered floor cleaner and 2 quarts of water. (If you prefer Metric measures, use 200ml of liquid ammonia, 50ml of powdered floor cleaner and 2 litres of water.)

Apply this solution to a small area of the floor (about 4 square feet), let it stand for several minutes to break up the polymer, then scrub with #0000 steel wool and rinse off.

If the polish buildup on your floor is a paste wax, however, it should be removed with petroleum solvent or mineral spirits. Make sure the room is well ventilated.

HEEL MARKS ON NO-WAX FLOOR

I have a no-wax vinyl floor and would like to know how to remove black heel marks from it without damaging the built-in shine.

The term no-wax is now being applied to two different kinds on vinyl flooring. One has a wet look finish (actually polyurethane) and an orange-skin texture. The other is a pure vinyl

with a very smooth, high gloss surface. If you have the first kind you can remove the heel marks with one of the general purpose liquid household cleaners. Apply with a soft cloth and rub firmly. If you have a pure vinyl flooring, the marks can be removed easily and safely with a little *white* paste wax. Apply with a soft cloth and rub firmly. If you are not sure which type of no-wax flooring you have, contact the supplier and ask for the manufacturer's maintenace instructions.

URETHANE FINISH PEELING

Our hardwood floor had a high-gloss urethane finish that we decided last year to cover with a satin urethane finish. This looked fine for a few months but recently it has begun to peel off in a number of places. Could there have been something wrong with this finish or did we apply it incorrectly?

You applied it incorrectly, I'm afraid. No finish sticks very well to a glossy surface, but urethane is particularly sensitive to this problem. You should have sanded the floor lightly with #80 or #100 paper or #0000 steel wool to remove the shine and provide a "tooth" for the new finish. All you can do now is sand off the remaining satin finish, which otherwise will continue to peel. Even better, remove the finish entirely and start again.

VINYL FLOOR BUCKLED

We had sheet vinyl flooring put down over the old wood floor in our kitchen. Quarter-inch plywood was applied first – to provide a smooth surface, the workers told me. This was nailed to the old floor, then the sheet vinyl was applied with adhesive. That was done in the winter time and it looked fine for awhile, but now the floor has started to buckle. The flooring company says they did their part of the job correctly and the problem must be in the old wood floor. What do you think?

I think they laid the plywood too tightly. The air in your house was probably very dry when they put the underlayment down during the winter. Now that the humidity has increased the plywood is expanding and can do nothing but buckle. The proper way to apply the plywood is to leave a gap of 1/16 in. to 1/8 in. on all edges. Also, it should be fastened with 1 1/4 in. ringed flooring nails every 6 in. around the edges and every 12 in. across the face. The only way to correct the problem now is to remove the flooring and underlayment and start again.

PATCHING SHEET VINYL

I burned a pot and as I was lifting it from the stove, part of it fell off and burned a hole in the sheet vinyl floor. Is there any way I can repair this without having to replace the flooring?

You can patch the floor with a piece of the same material. If you don't have a spare piece lying around you can cut one out of the floor under the refrigerator. You'll need a piece a few inches larger than the hole. Lay this over the hole, matching the pattern carefully. Tape it to the floor with masking tape, then use a metal straightedge and a razor knife to cut out a more-or-less square patch section around the hole. Make each cut several times to cut through both thicknesses of flooring.

Remove the taped section and then pry up and remove the piece that was burned. Apply linoleum cement to the matching patch and press it in place. Wipe off any excess adhesive, then cover the patch with a flat board and a heavy weight until the adhesive has set.

POLISHING A VINYL FLOOR

We have just had a very expensive, pure vinyl floor put down in our kitchen and I would like to know the proper way to care for it and what kind of polish to use.

Dust it regularly and wash it when necessary with a mop or sponge moistened with warm water plus a little mild sink detergent. Rinse with clean water and vinegar - about one ounce to a quart of water. This will cut the soap film and prevent streaking.

The best way to maintain a high shine on pure vinyl is to buff it regularly with an electric floor polisher fitted with lambswool pads. Move the polisher very slowly, allowing the friction of the pads to warm the surface of the vinyl. This softens it just enough to let the polisher buff out fine scratches or wear marks and restore the shine. Even heavily used floors treated this way will keep a high shine for many years of service. Polishes are not required.

REMOVING VINYL TILES

I would like to lay one of the do-it-yourself sheet vinyl flooring materials in my kitchen. What is the best way to remove the old vinyl tiles?

Most manufacturers do not recommend removing either sheet or tile flooring. This can be very difficult to do, in any case, and may leave a rough surface that will show through the new flooring. If the present flooring is smooth and firmly attached, the new material can simply be applied on top of it. If it is loose or curled it should be fastened down with 1 ¼ in. ringed flooring nails. Gaps or holes can be filled and levelled with a plaster patching compound or similar material.

But if the floor is in very bad shape, the best thing to do is cover it with ¼ in. (6mm) plywood, good-one-side (G1S) or underlayment grade. Particleboard and chipboard are not recommended. The panels should be laid with staggered joints left open ⅟₆₄ in. to allow for expansion, and fastened with 1 ¼ in. flooring nails every 6 in. around the edges and every 12 in. across the face. New flooring should then be applied according to the manufacturer's instructions.

SEAMS CURLED ON VINYL FLOOR

We had a new sheet vinyl floor laid in our kitchen about a year ago, and now the seams have opened and curled, allowing water and dirt to get underneath. How can we repair this?

The flooring job could not have been done properly, and the problem should have been reported to the applicator as soon as it appeared. The best way to make seam joints in sheet vinyl flooring, after the edges have been cut to fit exactly, is to apply an epoxy adhesive under both sides of the seam and use a special solvent-type seam sealer to weld the edges together permanently. I suggest you ask the flooring company to send an expert to correct the problem.

REMOVING SHEET VINYL

We have just bought a house with hardwood floors in the living room, dining room and hall that have been covered with sheet vinyl, firmly glued in place. How can we take it off so we can have the floors refinished?

Use a razor knife to cut the vinyl wear surface into narrow strips, which can then be pulled away from the fibre backing. Be careful not to cut through to the hardwood floor. Try a strip about 12 in. wide first to see if this can be pulled off without difficulty. Rolling it around a rolling pin or a bottle may help you apply even pressure. If necessary, cut in narrower strips.

Then use a broad putty knife to scrape the fibre backing off the floor. This should come off fairly easily; if not, rent or borrow an industrial hot air gun to soften the adhesive. It is advisable to wear a dust mask when doing this, since the fibre backing used on most sheet vinyl flooring contains asbestos fibres. The hardwood flooring will have to be sanded and refinished, of course.

STREAKY VINYL

I have been polishing the vinyl floor in my kitchen with a solvent-based liquid wax for several years, and recently switched to an acrylic floor polish, but I can't get this to go on smoothly. It looks streaky and dull in places. Am I doing something wrong?

Water-based acrylic floor polishes do not adhere very well to a waxed surface. The rule is that you can apply a solvent-based polish over a water-based polish, but you can't do it the other way around.

The two different polishes will have to be removed separately. A solution of 1 cup of liquid ammonia and ¼ cup of powdered floor cleaner to 2 quarts of water will remove the acrylic polish. The wax finish can be removed with petroleum solvent such as Varsol. Both solutions should be applied with a pad of very fine steel wool (#0000). Petroleum solvent is flammable, so make sure the room is well ventilated and don't allow any open flames. When both polishes have been removed you will find that the acrylic polish will go on without any trouble.

VARNISH ON VINYL TILES

We recently bought an older house that is in very good condition except for what appears to be a heavy buildup of wax on the kitchen floor tiles. None of the commercial floor strippers seem to work, even with strenuous scrubbing. Is there something stronger I can use?

Commercial strippers made for use on vinyl or vinyl-asbestos tiles should do the job if it is really a buildup of floor polish. Try doubling the recommended strength and applying it with #0000 steel wool.

I suspect, however, that the previous owner has mistakenly applied urethane or varnish to the vinyl floor in an attempt to give it a permanent shine. Paint remover can be used to take this off, but do just a small area at a time – no more than four tiles – and make sure the room is well ventilated. Use a pad of burlap or steel wool, not a metal scraper, to remove the softened finish.

Flooring manufacturers don't recommend this treatment, but I have tested a number of different kinds of paint remover on several brands of floor tile and found that none of them were harmed. To be on the safe side, however, test one tile in an inconspicuous spot.

VINYL FLOOR HAS YELLOWED

The white vinyl on our kitchen floor has turned yellow in the area where I stand in front of the sink. What causes this? Is there anything I can use to remove the stain? Regular cleaners don't work.

The fact that the discoloration is most noticeable where you stand suggests that it comes from the soles of your shoes. Rubber soles, for instance, sometimes contain chemicals that stain vinyl, but plastic soles can also do it. (Floor mats of these materials can stain vinyl, too.)

Another possible source of the stain is an asphalt driveway, particularly a new one. But even an old driveway will transfer enough bitumen to the soles of your shoes to make a noticeable stain on a white vinyl floor after a few years. (The Japanese custom of exchanging your shoes for slippers at the door makes a lot of sense.)

Unfortunately, most of these stains are very difficult to remove once they have penetrated the surface of the vinyl. The use of fine steel wool (#0000) and a heavy-duty cleaning solution will sometimes work, however. So will a strong solution of chlorine laundry bleach - say one part to four parts water. A petroleum solvent such as Varsol is also safe to use on vinyl if the room is well ventilated.

WAX BUILDUP ON OAK FLOOR

How can I remove a heavy wax buildup from a hardwood floor? The only wax strippers I can find all say they should NOT be used on wood floors.

Most wax removers are water-based solutions made for use on vinyl flooring, and as a general rule the use of water on wood floors should be avoided. Petroleum solvents or mineral spirits such as Varsol and Shellsol, or any of the paint *thinners* that are sold at hardware stores can all be used to remove wax buildup from wood floors. To avoid a streaky finish, use a number of clean cloths and discard each one when it gets dirty. These solvents are inflammable, however, so leave doors and windows open for good ventilation.

WAX BUILDUP ON VINYL

I recently moved into a house that has a heavy buildup of wax or other polish on the vinyl floor. I've tried using a strong ammonia solution but this does not seem to take it all off. If there anything stronger I can use?

The standard formula for a floor polish remover is one cup of liquid household ammonia and a quarter cup of powdered floor cleaner or dishwasher detergent to two quarts of water, but for tough jobs it is better to double or even triple the amount of ammonia. (Use with plenty of ventilation.)

A solvent that is much better than ammonia for removing modern acrylic floor polishes (very few actually contain wax anymore) is a chemical with the impressive name of monoethanolamine, which you will find listed on the label of some "wax strippers" sold at supermarkets.

Another trick is to let the solution soak into the old polish for at least three minutes before scrubbing it off with a nylon scrubbing pad. A little extra soaking time will make the job a lot easier. Do a small area at a time - say 2 ft x 2 ft - and wipe up the dissolved polish before going on to the next area. Finally, rinse the floor with a good sponge mop and *several changes of clean water* to avoid leaving streaks on the vinyl floor.

FURNITURE CARE

ALLIGATORED FURNITURE FINISH

A small table in our living room has been standing for a long time beside a window, and now the finish has developed a pattern of fine cracks that resemble alligator skin. Is there any way I can restore this without removing the entire finish?

This is probably a lacquer finish, in which case the remedy is fairly simple. Simply brush a generous application of lacquer thinner on the tabletop and let it stand for two or three minutes, then brush again to smooth out the softened lacquer just as if you were applying a new finish - which, in effect, you are.

Test the lacquer thinner first to make sure it will dissolve the finish. If it doesn't, then you have a varnish finish that can only be taken off

CIGARETTE BURN ON TABLE

After a recent party at our house I discovered a cigarette burn on my dining table. Is there any way I can remove this without have the whole table refinished?

If it's a valuable piece, the best thing to do is call in a professional with the skill and special materials needed to make an invisible repair, and do it right in your house. Most furniture stores can give you the name of someone who does this work. Or look in the Yellow Pages under FURNITURE REPAIRING & REFINISHING.

If you'd like to do it yourself, used the curved tip of a knife blade to scrape off the damaged finish and any charred wood underneath. A very shallow scar can be touched up with a matching colored lacquer that comes in a small bottle with a brush-cap, like nail polish, available at most hardware stores. Deeper scars can be filled with a matching crayon or wax stick. Hold it against a hot knife blade and drop the melting wax into the depression. When the wax hardens, scrape the excess off carefully with a razor blade, then rub the surface lightly with your finger to blend the edge of the patch into the rest of the finish.

FURNITURE TOO DRY?

I have removed the paint from an old dresser made of oak, and have found that the wood is so dry that it is beginning to crack. How can I get the vital moisture into the wood, and what finish should I use to keep it there?

Many people have the impression that wood contains "natural juices" that must be retained to preserve its vitality. This is nonsense. The finest furniture woods are kiln dried to a moisture content of only 6% to 8%, which is a lot drier than the air in our homes. And no matter how it is finished, wood will continue to absorb moisture until it approaches the humidity level of the air around it. Good furniture will contain more moisture than when it was made, in other words.

If the furniture was made of improperly dried wood, however, it will crack or check as it reaches the lower humidity level of our houses (particularly in winter). There is no finish that will prevent this. The only way you can add moisture to the wood is to raise the humidity in your house, and that may just cause other problems.

GLASS TABLETOP SCRATCHED

After a large dinner party we noticed a scratch in the top of our smoked glass dining table. While it is possible to turn the top over, the scratch is still very visible. Is there anything we can use to grind out the scratch or fill it? Is there a wax or polish that will keep the glass from being scratched like this again?

It takes special equipment and abrasives to grind and repolish glass, but you'll find firms that do this work listed in the Yellow Pages. A less expensive remedy is to fill the scratch with several layers of one of the acrylic floor polishes, such as Future or Durashine. Apply it to the scratch with a toothpick and let each coat dry before adding another. Keep building it up until it is even with the surface. Use a razor blade to scrape off any excess. This should make the scratch just about invisible.

There is no wax or polish that will keep the glass from being scratched by hard, sharp objects. The best protection is to use table mats under everything.

IMPORTED FURNITURE DRYING OUT

Eight years ago I bought a carved walnut coffee table in India and brought it back to Canada. I have never oiled it, and now the wood has dried to a lighter color and has started to crack in a few places. What kind of oil should I use to restore the color and prevent the wood from drying out any more? (We have a humidifier, incidentally.)

To restore the color, apply teak oil, one of the Danish oil finishes, or equal parts of boiled linseed oil and petroleum solvent or turpentine. These should just be wiped on, allowed to sink in for 15 minutes or so, then wiped off with a dry cloth. Repeat in six months.

But there is no treatment or finish that will prevent the wood from drying out and cracking. Even with a humidifier, winter air in your home will sometimes be much drier than it is where this piece of furniture was made. That causes no problems in their climate, but when the furniture gets here it begins to dry out to our humidity level, and usually cracks in the process. One easy way to raise the humidity level in your home during the winter is to reduce the air leakage with weatherstripping and caulking. It is the influx of relatively dry winter air that lowers the humidity in our homes (and wastes heat, too, of course),

CARE OF OAK CUPBOARDS

We have a new home with beautifully finished oak cupboards and cabinets in the kitchen. What should I use to preserve them?

Just dust them when necessary and wipe them occasionally with a damp cloth or sponge. A couple of drops of sink detergent or one of the liquid household cleaners can be used to remove finger marks or grease spots. The factory finish on the wood is tougher and more durable than any wax or polish you could apply, and such treatment is unnecessary. Excessive use of waxes and polishes is the main cause of problems with furniture finishes, in fact. Relax and enjoy.

OIL FINISH SCRATCHED

We applied a natural Danish oil finish to our mahogany doors. One of them was scratched recently, and where I applied more Danish oil to the mark it turned very dark and is more noticable than ever. What is the proper way to remove such marks?

The broken wood fibres left in the scratch soak up the oil and become darker than the solid wood around them. Scratches must be filled or sanded smooth before the oil is applied.

OILY TABLE

Some years ago we had a walnut coffee table with an oil finish made for us. We started putting oil on it regularly to maintain the finish, and have had to do this fairly often because papers placed on the table soak up the oil and leave a white area on the wood. Is there something we can put on to prevent this happening?

It sounds as if you have been using the wrong kind of oil. You are supposed to use a thinned "drying oil" such as linseed or tung, generally sold as Teak Oil. These dry hard within a day or two and could not be absorbed into a piece of paper left on the surface after that. You have probably been using a light machine oil of some kind. This never dries. Remove the oil with petroleum solvent or paint thinner, then wipe with Teak Oil, allow it to stand for about 20 minutes, and wipe off with a dry cloth. Such a treatment should not be necessary more than once a year.

SHINY PATCHES ON FURNITURE FINISH

Several years ago we purchased a walnut bedroom suite that had a dull, natural wood finish. The instructions that came with it said not to use wax or other polish and to clean it only with a soft cloth moistened with lukewarm water and a drop of detergent. Over the years the finish has become shiny in spots, particularly around the drawer handles, and these areas are not restored by the soap and water treatment. I'm afraid to try anything else. What can I do to restore the finish?

That was good advice and it applies to any furniture finish. The shiny spots may have two causes; oil from your fingers, and the constant rubbing of the finish over the years. A cloth lightly dampened with Varsol or other petroleum solvent will remove the oil. If a shine remains, rub the area with number #0000 steel wool to dull it slightly.

CARE OF TEAK FURNITURE

I have just purchased a high-quality teak table and would like to know the proper way to take care of it.

I assume that you like the distinctive color and grain pattern and want to maintain the natural, open-textured finish that is characteristic of fine teak furniture. The reason I mention this is that most of the advice you get on the care of teak will change all of these attractive features.

Most people will tell you, for instance, that you have to rub the table with teak oil every few weeks "to keep the wood from drying out". In less than a year this treatment will build up a varnish-like layer of linseed oil that gives the wood a dark amber tone and fills the open grain. The color and texture of the teak furniture you bought will be completly changed.

Like other kiln-dried furniture woods, teak contains far less moisture than it will be exposed to in your home, so it's not going to "dry out". The penetrating oil-resin finish that is applied at the factory doesn't dry out, either, although it will deteriorate if it is exposed to direct sunlight too long.

So the first thing to realize is that teak, like other furniture, requires very little attention. Excessive use of sprays, creams, pastes, oils or other polishes is the cause of most furniture care problems. Teak should be dusted regularly (a little lemon oil on the cloth will help pick up dust) and wiped occasionally with a damp sponge. A drop of dish detergent on the sponge will help remove finger marks and other grease spots.

If you feel guilty because you're not doing more for your furniture, you can rub it down once a year with teak oil and a pad of #0000 steel wool, then buff with a clean, dry cloth. (Don't let the oil sit on the surface for more than 15 minutes or it will become sticky.)

And don't be fooled by claims about "rejuvenating the wood" or "restoring the natural oils" with various polishes. Such claims are about as valid as those once made for snake oil medicines.

RESTORING A TEAK TABLE

Our teak dining table has served us well for many years, but it is now showing a few light and dark patches from food spills, hot dishes, water marks and general wear, I guess. Is there any way to restore the tabletop without having to refinish it entirely?

Use a cloth moistened with petroleum solvent (Varsol, Shellsol, etc.) to remove dirt, oil stains and wax or other polish, then rub the surface in the direction of the grain with very fine steel wool (#0000) until you achieve a soft, even, satin sheen overall. This will remove most of the heat spots and water rings, but a little extra rubbing may be necessary on some of them. Any light patches that remain can be darkened by wiping them with a cloth dipped in a maple or teak wood stain. Rub the stain into the wood, then remove any surplus with a soft cloth. If a darker color is required to match the rest of the finish, let the first application dry and then re-apply. If it is too dark, rub with steel wool.

Finally, wipe the entire table with a commercial teak oil or a mixture of one part boiled linseed oil to two parts petroleum solvent. Leave this for about 30 minutes, touching up any dry spots that appear, then remove all surplus oil with a soft cloth. Don't use the table for several hours.

TUNG OIL OVER OLD FINISH

I tried refinishing my coffee table by removing all the wax with petroleum solvent and then applying two coats of something called tung oil, which the salesman said would make an excellent finish. Unfortunately, it didn't work out that way. The new finish is sticky, attracts dust and is difficult to clean. How can I remove this and restore the original finish?

Tung oil is similar to linseed oil, and neither of them should be applied to an existing finish in this way. They must be diluted first with turpentine or paint thinner, applied with a cloth, then wiped off with a dry cloth after about 15 minutes, leaving the merest suggestion of oil on the surface. They should never be brushed on like varnish and left to dry - because they don't harden properly this way, as you've discovered.

The tung oil will have hardened by now as much as it's going to, however, and the only thing that will take it off is paint remover, which will also take off the original finish, of course. For a new finish I suggest at least two coats of satin urethane varnish.

VENEER LIFTING

In one small area of our walnut dining table the veneer is beginning to bubble and crack. Can you tell me what causes this and how to repair it?

It is either caused by the table getting wet or by direct sunlight falling on it for a long period. Use a hypodermic syringe oiler (available at any hobby shop) to inject one of the white resin adhesives under the raised veneer. If necessary, use a razor knife to slit the veneer bubble along a grain line, and then inject adhesive under both edges. Press the veneer down to squeeze out any surplus; wipe this off with a damp cloth or sponge. Then cover the area with a piece of polyethylene film (which won't stick to the adhesive), place a flat board on top and apply a heavy weight such as a concrete block. Remove after 24 hours and rub the repaired area with #0000 steel wool and a little lemon oil.

WATER SPOTS ON TABLE

I have a walnut veneer table that has been damaged by water spills from the potted plants we have placed on it. This has left light-colored spots that are rough and cracked along the grain of the wood. Is there any way I can restore the top without having to refinish it entirely?

Smooth the rough spots with #0000 steel wool, then rub them with a light walnut furniture stain and remove the surplus with a soft cloth. If a darker tone is needed, apply more stain. When dry, apply paste wax and buff to restore the gloss.

WHITE HAZE ON FURNITURE FINISH

Do you know of anything that will remove a white haze that has developed on a modern solid maple table? I think it may have been caused by mixing different kinds of furniture polish or using a damp cloth occasionally to clean the surface.

The occasional use of a damp cloth will not harm any furniture finish, so it can't be that. Mixing polishes will sometimes cause a white or bluish haze to develop on the surface, but this can usually be removed by using several clean cloths moistened with a petroleum solvent such as Varsol. If this does not remove the haze, I suggest you try automobile rubbing compound, a gentle abrasive paste that is used for smoothing and polishing autobody finishes. You can get it at any auto supply store and most hardware stores. Apply with a damp cloth, rubbing in the direction of the grain. If this dulls the finish slightly, apply paste wax and buff to restore the gloss.

HEATING

CLOSING ROOMS TO CONSERVE HEAT

Two of our bedrooms upstairs are not used, so to conserve heat we turned the heat off to these rooms and shut the doors. Now we've noticed that these rooms smell musty, the walls are damp and there are black spots on the ceiling. What causes this and what can we do about it?

Condensation on the cold walls and ceiling in the unheated rooms has encouraged the growth of mildew. This may also develop in clothing, mattresses and bedding left in those rooms. Dampness is the inevitable result of lowering the temperature in these rooms, and this is why it is not a good idea to close off part of a house to save heat. It will be less expensive in the long run if you heat these rooms and leave the doors open for ventilation.

KEROSENE vs STOVE OIL

I have a portable kerosene heater that I use to supplement my electric heating. Is it true that I can use Number One stove oil in it in place of kerosene?

No. The Canadian Standards Association (CSA) specifies the use of high grade (#1K) pure white kerosene only. Stove oil is a little heavier or thicker than kerosene, produces more smoke and odor, and can clog up the ceramic wick used in these portable heaters.

TAR DRIPPING FROM FURNACE VENT

I have been doing some furniture stripping and refinishing in my basement this winter, and recently noticed a tar-like substance dripping out around the bottom of my gas furnace vent pipe. Can you tell me what is causing this?

It is very unlikely that this is tar, but there is a simple test. If the substance can be removed with a wet cloth, it is neither tar not asphalt, but what gas industry experts identify as a thick solution of iron chloride produced by corrosion inside the metal vent pipe. This is almost certainly caused, they tell me, by the methylene chloride vapors from the paint remover. These heavy vapors fall to the floor and are drawn into the furnace, where they are broken down by heat and combine with water vapor in the flue gases to produce a very strong, corrosive solution of hydrochloric acid.

U.S. studies have found that even minute quantities of such chlorine-based solvents in the air, too low to be detected by smell or hazardous to health, can cause serious corrosion to gas furnace ventpipes, oil or gas furnace heat exchangers, and even to the heating elements in an electric furnace. The problem has been recognized for years in industrial plants using chlorine-based solvents, and a number of articles about it have appeared in technical journals, but little attention has been paid to the risk of damage in home furnaces. This is partly because such solvents (chemists call them chlorinated hydrocarbons) were once rarely used around the house, but they have become much more common in recent years. In addition to methylene chloride paint removers, they include two popular nonflammable solvents, tri- and per-chloroethylene, that are sold as home drycleaning fluids and also used as solvents in some flooring adhesives.

Such products generally carry warning labels about the need for good ventilation, but most people think this just means opening a nearby window a bit. The trouble is, we are sealing our houses much tighter these days and have far less ventilation than we think we have, particularly in the winter months. Information I have learned in researching this answer, however, convinces me that paint removers, "chloro" cleaning fluids and flooring adhesives labelled as containing these solvents should be used *very* sparingly during the winter months because of possible corrosion damage to the heating system - and also, of course, because the fumes can be hazardous to health, anyway, in confined areas.

I suggest that you save your paint removing until the heating season is over, and then have your gas furnace and vent pipe inspected to assess the extent of the present corrosion.

DOES THERMOSTAT SETBACK SAVE HEAT?

My wife says we could lower our heating costs if we replace our thermostat with one that will set the temperature back at night automatically and turn it up again before we get up. I don't see how this can do any good. Won't it take just as much fuel to get the house back up to temperature again?

Consider this: If you turned the heat down in your house while you were away for a week, then turned it up again when you got home, would you save money? Of course. Would you use less fuel if you turned it down for two days? Certainly, but not as much, of course. A cooler house always uses less heat, even if it is just for a few hours.

The amount you save will depend on the outside temperature, the length of the setback period and its *average* temperature. The latter depends on how long it takes your house to cool down to the setback temperature and your heating system to warm it up again, but it will always be lower than the regular thermostat setting, so you will always save *some* heat by turning the thermostat down.

In the average home you will reduce your heating costs by about 2% for each degree Celsius the house temperature is lowered for an 8-hour period (1% for each degree fahrenheit). If you set the thermostat back 5°C (9°F) overnight, for instance, you will reduce your heating costs around 10%. And if you also turn the heat down during the day while everyone is away, you will make a further saving, but not quite as much because of the higher outdoor temperature and the free heat supplied by sunlight.

CONVERTING BACK TO COAL

I have an old coal furnace that was converted to oil many years ago. Oil is expensive now and natural gas is not available in our area, so I was wondering if I could reduce my heating bills by switching back to coal.

For a given amount of delivered heat, coal is now about 25% cheaper than fuel oil. But it is a lot more work, don't forget, and your old coal furnace cannot be controlled by a central thermostat. There is another problem, too. The cast iron grates that support the coal in the firebox were probably thrown away years ago, and the furnace cannot be converted back to coal without them. I am told it is just about impossible to get new grates for these old coal furnaces.

BASEBOARD HEATER KEEPS CYCLING

One of the electric baseboard heaters in our living room keeps cycling on and off, even though the room temperature is not up to the wall thermostat setting.

Something may be blocking the circulation of air through the baseboard heater, causing it to overheat and trip the safety device that shuts the current off. Check to see if the drapes, carpet, furniture, or anything else is touching the heater. Also remove the front panel (it pulls out at the bottom and then lifts off) to find out if something has fallen into the baseboard unit.

If there is nothing blocking the air flow through the baseboard, there may be something wrong with the safety cutoff switch. You'll have to ask an electrician to check and replace this.

DRAPES DISCOLORED OVER BASEBOARD HEATERS

The electric baseboard heaters we installed this winter have made the white drapes and curtains above them turn yellow. Why is this happening?

Baseboard heaters draw cool air from the floor, heat it, and circulate it upwards into the room. If some of this air passes through the drapes and curtains, they will trap any dirt in it just as a filter would.

The baseboard heaters produce no dirt themselves, so it must come from the room itself. Dust can be picked up from the floor or carpet, or from the air circulating in the room. But if the white fabric is turning yellow, the most likely cause is tobacco smoke. This is certainly the case if there are any heavy smokers in the house. Over an extended period, even moderate smoking will do this.

SAFETY OF BASEBOARD HEATERS

I have winterized my summer cottage and installed a 2500-watt baseboard heater. What worries me, however, is that the heater is applied directly to plywood wall panelling. Is this a fire hazard? Shouldn't some insulating material be placed between the heating unit and the wall?

All baseboard heaters sold in Canada must meet CSA standards that permit direct application to any conventional wall panelling material.

CLOSE UNUSED DUCTWORK?

We recently converted from an oil-fired warm air heating system to electric baseboard heating. We keep the basement fairly cool (about 45°F) and we are wondering if we should close off all the floor ducts to keep the cool air from coming upstairs during the heating season.

The air won't circulate through your heating ducts unless you turn the furnace fan on. But most old warm air systems don't have a cold air return duct in the basement, anyway.

You are most likely to have cold floors upstairs because of the very low temperature you are maintaining in the basement. A better way to save heat is to insulate the basement walls. This will allow you to raise the termperature down there, which will keep the floors warmer and require less heat upstairs.

ELECTRIC HOT WATER HEATING

We have oil-fired hot water heating in our house and would like to convert it to electricity. Is there an electrical element that can be inserted in the furnace to heat the water?

No, but you can replace the furnace with an electric water heater that is only 2 feet square, 9 in. thick and simply hangs on the wall. You will also need a 200-amp electrical service, however.

OUTSIDE AIR SUPPLY

I understand that my gas furnace draws a lot of warm air out of the house and up the chimney. Will it save any heat if I enclose the furnace in an insulated room with a direct air vent to the outside? How much ventilation must I have in this room?

This can be done but it won't save much money. Only about 3% of your heat is lost in the air that is drawn up the gas vent, and this ventilation is needed, anyway, to control humidity and odors in the house. Also, heat will be lost from the furnace and ductwork in the cold furnace room, reducing the amount of heat the furnace delivers to the house.

In short, it's not a very good idea. But to answer your second question, you would need a 5 in. diameter outside air duct terminating within 12 in. above and 24 in. horizontally from the burner level of the furnace. The duct should be shielded and screened on the outside, but must not contain a manual damper.

TESTING FURNACE AIR SUPPLY

I have read stories about houses being so tightly sealed that poisonous combustion fumes from a gas furnace were drawn back into the house through the open draft hood. How can I tell if I have enough ventilation to prevent this?

I should point out first that the combustion fumes from a gas furnace are normally no more poisonous than the hot air that rises from a gas stove. Only under very rare conditions is toxic carbon monoxide produced. Secondly, even a moderately well sealed house has enough air leakage and other ventilation to change all the air in the house *every two hours*, according to National Research Council studies, and this is considerably more air than the average gas furnace needs.

The problem you refer to occurs not because the house is too tightly sealed, but because other appliances in the house are drawing air out of it much more powerfully then the furnace is. A briskly burning open fireplace, for instance, uses ten times as much air as the average gas furnace. Even a kitchen exhaust fan will draw four times as much air out of the house as a gas furnace uses, and a clothes dryer takes about the same.

There are times when this demand on the air supply will create a partial vacuum in the house that draws air *down* the gas vent, causing the furnace combustion fumes to spill into the house, and sometimes this can cause serious problems. To find out if your gas furnace is getting all the air it needs, turn the thermostat down to shut off the furnace, then wait 10 minutes before conducting the following test. If you have a fireplace, light it and get it going well, then close all the windows and doors and turn on the clothes dryer and any other exhaust fans you have. If the fireplace begins to smoke, this is one indication that the house is not getting enough air. Next turn up the room thermostat to start the furnace, then hold a lighted match in front of the open draft hood on the front of the furnace. (If you have a gas-fired boiler instead of a warm air furnace, the draft hood will be located in the vent pipe on top of the boiler.)

The match flame should be drawn *into* the draft opening, indicating that the air is going up the vent as it should. If the flame is blown *away* from the draft opening, however, you have a potentially dangerous situation. The remedy is simple; just make sure that the furnace room has an adequate supply of outside air at all times. Blocking a nearby window slightly open is one easy way to do it. Another is to install a 4 in. or 5 in. diameter duct bringing outside air to within one foot of the furnace air intake. To keep cold air from coming in the vent when it is not needed, a Canadian-made unit is available that has an automatic damper that opens only when the furnace is on. This device has been approved by the Canadian Gas Association and can be installed by any licensed serviceman.

DOES IT PAY TO TURN THE PILOT LIGHT OFF?

We have a conventional gas furnace. Would it pay us to turn the pilot light off for the summer?

It might. The average pilot light uses about 570 cubic feet or 16 cubic metres of natural gas a month, and your gas company can tell you how much that costs. But if you do not use gas for anything else - cooking or a water heater, for instance - then you won't save very much money because you will be billed the minimum monthly charge, anyway.

If you have other gas appliances besides the furnace, however, then you will save the full value of the gas the pilot light uses. But you will have to turn the pilot light on again yourself when the heating season comes. (Instructions are usually printed on the furnace.) If you have to call in a serviceman to do it, this will cost enough to wipe out most of the saving.

AIR IN RADIATORS

We have a hot water heating system with old-fashioned cast iron radiators. Three years ago we replaced the oil-fired boiler with an electric boiler and water pump. Since then we have had trouble with air collecting in the upstairs radiators. If we don't bleed the air out of these regularly the water won't circulate properly. We were told this would stop after all the air was taken out, but the problem persists.

The water temperature may be set too high. The system was probably designed for a temperature of around 65°C (150°F), but modern boilers are usually set much higher. Lowering the temperature setting on the aquastat should reduce the problem. Some air will still collect in the upper radiators occasionally, but you can install float valves on the radiators to get rid of this automatically.

ENCLOSING A RADIATOR

We have a hot water heating system with a lot of old-fashioned cast iron radiators. Would there be any fire hazard if we had wooden enclosures put around them to make them look a little more attractive? These would include perforated metal screens to let the air through.

There is no danger of a fire - radiators don't get hot enough for that - but the enclosures will interfere with the circulation of air over the radiators and therefore reduce the amount of heat they give off. This might not cause any serious problems, but I don't think it's a very good idea.

HEATING WITH HARD WATER

We live in an area where the water is very hard and we heat our house with a hot water system - boiler, pump and baseboard radiators. A buildup of lime deposit in the pipes is causing trouble with the pump, according to our serviceman, and I would like to know what we can put in the water to soften it and prevent further problems. We drain the water and replace it every two or three years.

There's no need to add anything to the water, nor should it be changed. When the heating system is first filled, any calcium in the water will be deposited on the boiler pipes within a few weeks in the form of a very thin layer that causes no trouble at all. From then on the water is effectively softened and no further lime buildup can occur - unless you add fresh hard water to the system, as you have been doing.

HOUSE OVERHEATING

We had a circulating pump added to our gravity hot water heating system to improve the heat distribution, but now it's working too well. The house temperature sometimes rises above the thermostat setting.

Most likely this is caused by the water temperature being set too high. Modern hydronic heating systems generally use a setting of 170° to 180°F (77° to 82°C), but cast iron radiators absorb so much heat at this temperature that they continue to warm the room long after the burner has shut off. You should lower the setting on your aquastat to the water temperature the pipes and radiators were designed for - between 140° and 160°F (60° to 71°C).

KEEPING PIPES FROM RUSTING

We have a hot water heating system with galvanized pipes, and we haven't changed the water in it since we bought the house four years ago. Will you please tell me how to do this? We are concerned about the iron pipes rusting.

That's one maintenance job you can forget about. The old water is a lot better for the boiler and pipes than new water would be. That's because it is the oxygen that is dissolved in the fresh water that causes iron to rust. Once the oxygen is used up (in a few months, at most) no further rusting will take place. The same goes for any hardness chemicals that would be deposited inside the pipes; there are none left in the water you have there now.

BOILER PUMP RUNS CONSTANTLY

We have a hot water heating system, and a couple of years ago we switched from oil to natural gas. Only recently did we realize that the circulating pump has been running constantly, 24 hours a day, winter and summer. The company that installed the new boiler says the pump is supposed to run all the time, but this doesn't sound right to me. Shouldn't it shut off automatically when no heat is required?

Although there are other ways of doing it, many residential heating systems use a circulating pump that runs continuously *during the heating season* while the thermostat controls the burner. The pump is not supposed to run all year, however. There should be a switch near the furnace that turns off the burner controls and the pump at the end of the heating season - and turns them on again, of course, when the season begins. The heating system operates automatically, but you still have to turn it on and off for the heating season.

TEMPERATURE SETBACK WITH HOT WATER HEATING

My house has an old hot water heating system. I was thinking of installing an automatic thermostat to set back the temperature at night, but the boiler serviceman says this won't save any money because it takes too long to bring water back up to temperature. Seems to me the same energy-saving principle would apply as with a warm air heating system.

You're right. Lowering the temperature of the house *for any period of time* will reduce its heat loss and lower fuel consumption. But you will have to set the DOWN and UP times a little earlier than you would if you had a warm air heating system, because water does take longer to cool down and warm up, and this means that you will not save as much money as you would with a warm air heating system.

The difference in the setback time will depend on the volume of water in the heating system and how fast it circulates. An old gravity system with a large boiler and pipes and slow circulation might require a couple of hours to get the house back up to temperature, but the time will be less if a circulating pump has been added. A modern hydronic system with small copper pipes and an instant boiler would rquire about the same time as a warm air system, perhaps as little as half an hour. Experience will show you the right setting.

UPGRADING A BOILER SYSTEM

We have recently bought an old house that is heated by a hot water boiler and cast iron radiators. We are thinking of converting the entire system to baseboard electric heating. Do you think this is a good idea?

Before you do this you should ask a plumbing/heating contractor to inspect your present system and advise you on its condition, what can be done to improve it and how much the work will cost. If all you need is a new boiler, for instance, it might pay you to put in an electric unit. These are very efficient and small enough to put on the wall.

Next, call in an electrical contractor for an estimate on installing electric baseboard heating throughout the house, then compare the cost of these two alternatives. But regardless of what type of electric heating you put in, you will also have the cost of upgrading your electrical service to 200 amps to carry this additional load - and this alone can run to $1500 or more. Get bids from at least three contractors before selecting one to upgrade your heating system.

DIRTY AIR FROM REGISTERS

We have a problem with our oil-fired, warm air heating system. The furnace is only five years old but the air coming from the room registers is very dirty and deposits a sooty, oily film on the walls and floors around them. We think there must be something wrong with the furnace, but the serviceman says it is working fine.

Oily soot can only come from the combustion gases, which means there must be a leak somewhere in the furnace that is allowing these to get into the warm air duct system. Rust holes are possible, but unlikely in a furnace this old. Most likely it is the result of poor servicing. When the serviceman cleans the furnace he must remove one or more access panels to get inside the heat exchanger. If these are not replaced very tightly, dirty combustion gases will leak into the warm air plenum and be carried through the duct system.

In furnaces that have what is called a "rear breech", the flue pipe passes through the cold air return plenum at the back of the furnace. A rusting pipe or loose connection here will also allow smoke to leak into the warm duct system. A good serviceman should be able to locate and correct any of these problems very quickly.

DUST FROM HEATING DUCTS

I have put three layers of cheesecloth over each of my heating registers and cold air return grilles in an effort to trap the dust we are getting upstairs from the furnace. This seems to have started since we added a wood-burning unit to our furnace. Will the cheesecloth have any effect on the operation of the furnace or the amount of heat we get?

Yes. The cheesecloth will reduce the amount of warm air being delivered to the rooms. This may be offset slightly by an increase in the temperature of the delivered air, but it will still mean that less heat is being extracted from the furnace and delivered to the rooms; more heat will be lost up the chimney, in other words.

This is a poor way to filter the air, anyway. There must be a filter in the furnace already, and this should be inspected regularly and cleaned or replaced whenever it is dirty. You can also buy a sticky solution to spray on the filter so it will catch dust particles that might pass through an untreated filter. This is sold at most stores that sell furnace filters. Or you can install an electrostatic air filter that will do an even better job of removing fine particles from the air.

I must point out, however, that the dust does not come from the furnace itself, as you suggest. All the combustion gases go up the chimney; they cannot mix with the air that is circulating through the ductwork. The dust originates in the house, but it might be coming from the firewood that presumably is being stored and handled in the basement. The cold air return intake in the basement could be picking this up and circulating it through the house.

FURNACE FAN RACES

Our warm air furnace makes a whirring noise like a racing motor for about 10 seconds before the air begins to come out of the registers.

It sounds like a loose fan belt. This is supposed to be slack enough to slip a little when the motor starts, to avoid putting a strain on the motor, but if the belt is too loose the motor will race for a time until the fan begins to turn. (And if it gets any looser, the fan won't turn at all.)

Check this by removing the access panel on the furnace and watching as someone turns up the thermostat. The fan motor will start about a minute after the burner comes on. If it races before the fan turns, switch off the furnace or open the circuit at the main service panel by removing the fuse or turning off the circuit-breaker, then tighten the fan belt with the adjustments provided on the motor mount. It should move no more than ¾ in. when you press it in the centre with your thumb.

COST OF RUNNING FURNACE FAN

Our furnace is equipped with an electronic air filter, which, because of health problems, we use all year. The furnace fan runs contantly and I would like to know if we could save electricity by switching it from manual to automatic control, and whether this can be done without harming the filter.

The average ¼ horsepower fan motor uses about 300 watts of electricity when it is running. If it is on constantly it will consume about 215 kilowatt hours (kwh) per month or 2600kwh a year. I don't know the exact rate you are paying for electricity, but at 4 ½ cents per kwh this works out to about $10 a month or $120 a year. The filter itself uses another $20 worth.

If the furnace fan is put on automatic control it probably will be on no more than 70% of the time during the heating season. This will only reduce your annual electricity bill by $21 (at the rate above), because you will still have to turn the fan on with the manual control during the summer months to keep the electronic filter working. Intermittant fan operation during the winter will not harm the filter because it is only on when the fan is running.

FURNACE FILTER vs HUMIDIFIER

I have a warm air furnace with a drum-type humidifier. I want to put in an electrostatic filter but someone told me this can't be used with a humidifier. Is this true?

As long as the humidifier is 12 in. or more from the filter, and is not located where water could drip on it, there should be no problem.

BAROMETRIC DAMPER ON WOOD FURNACE?

I heat a large house with a dual-fuel furnace that uses either wood or oil. There is a weighted, free-swinging damper in the furnace pipe. I would like to know if this is required for both fuels or just when oil is being used.

This is called a barometric damper, and its purpose is to maintain a steady draft pressure through the oil burner in spite of fluctuations in air pressure caused by weather changes. Although it is not needed for the wood-burning unit, it doesn't interfere with its operation. In any case, there is no practical way to use it only for one fuel. A special type of barometric damper that is not affected by creosote buildup should be used on dual-fuel furnaces like this.

FAN PROBLEM WITH WOOD FURNACE

We have a combination oil/wood furnace. It works fine on oil, but when we are burning wood the fan that circulates the warm air through the house doesn't come on until the air gets very hot.

There are two fan controls on your furnace; one on the oil burner side and one on the wood-burning side. The latter is not set correctly. Remove the cover from the fan control and hold the circular dial firmly with one hand while you move the FAN ON pointer to 120°F with the other (the pointer is probably set much higher than that now). The OFF pointer should be set at 90°F. These are also the recommended fan control settings for the oil burner side.

CLEANING WOOD STOVE DOOR

I have an airtight wood stove with a glass door that must be cleaned every day if I want to be able to see how the fire is burning. This means I have to let the fire go out, and one of the main advantages of an airtight stove is that I can close the draft door so the fire will burn slowly all day and use very little wood. How can I prevent the heavy brown deposit forming on the glass?

A smoldering fire causes the creosote deposit. A lot of people think an airtight stove should be shut down to burn very slowly all the time, but that creates a smoldering fire that produces a lot of smoke, tar and creosote. More serious than the dirty door is the creosote that is building up inside the chimney, because this can be a very serious fire hazard.

The stove must get enough air for the wood to burn properly, and the draft should be opened even more for about 10 minutes every hour to let the fire burn briskly and keep the chimney warm so that creosote deposits will not form. This will also help keep the glass door clean

I recommend using liquid drain cleaner to remove the creosote buildup from the glass. Two other cleaners have been suggested by a number of readers. One is wood ash applied with a damp cloth or sponge. The other is oven cleaner.

CREOSOTE PROBLEM

We used our wood stove all winter, and now there is a gummy deposit of creosote in the stovepipe and chimney. I tried one of the chemicals that was supposed to get rid of the creosote, but it didn't do any good. What should I use? A friend tells me we have been using the wrong kind of wood. Could this be true?

Any kind of wood will produce creosote if it's not burned correctly. A slow, smoldering fire with damp wood and too little draft is the most common cause of creosote buildup, but a cold, outside masonry chimney will also contribute to the problem. The remedy is to keep a hotter fire burning in the stove to warm the chimney. Just opening the draft for about 10 minutes every hour is usually enough to prevent the formation of creosote. A little experience will show you how much you need. Check the chimney with a mirror periodically.

I know of nothing that can be relied on to remove a buildup of creosote except a good cleaning by an expert, and I suggest you have this done as soon as possible to avoid a chimney fire.

GETTING HEAT TO FAR ROOMS

I have a 1600-square-foot, 2-year-old backs-plit house that is heated by a warm air furnace. I am having trouble getting heat to the rooms that are farthest from the furnace, even after I adjustd the dampers in the other ducts to force more air to the distant rooms. What I need, I think, is more air pressure from the furnace fan, which is belt-driven and has a ¼-horsepower motor. Should I put in a larger motor?

This may not be necessary. The speed of a belt-driven fan can be changed by adjusting the belt pulley on the motor. Turn the furnace off at the wall switch, remove the fan belt and loosen the setscrew that holds the outer half of the pulley on the motor shaft. Turn this part of the pulley one complete turn in a clockwise direction to close the gap and cause the fan belt to run higher in the groove, increasing the speed of the fan.

Tighten the pulley setscrew (it must rest on the flat side of the motor shaft), replace the fan belt and adjust the tension by moving the motor as required. There should be about ¾ in. play in the centre of the belt when you press it firmly. Turn the furnace on. If the fan speed is not high enough, repeat the process. The fan will be noisier with the increased speed, however, and this is usually the limiting factor.

HOT METAL SMELL FROM REGISTERS

We have a 19-year-old oil furnace and recently noticed that a "hot metal" smell is coming from the warm air registers every time the furnace comes on.

This could be due to a crack or hole in the firebrick lining of the combustion chamber, allowing the burner flame to reach the steel shell of the heat exchanger, on the other side of which the household air is circulating. You should have this checked immediately. Call your oil supplier.

NOISY FURNACE

Recently I purchased a modest bungalow in a quiet neighborhood. Normally you can hear a pin drop in the house, but when the furnace fan starts up it's like a pack of lions in the basement. The oil furnace is only five years old. There is no insulation in the basement ceiling. How can I soundproof the furnace?

First, find out why your furnace is making so much noise. It's a fairly recent model, after all, and shouldn't make this much noise. There are a number of things that could be wrong. The fan axle may be bent; the bearings may be defective; the fan mounting bolts may be loose; or the fan speed may be set too high. All of these are easily fixed. Call in a serviceman.

Soundproofing isn't very practical because much of the noise is carried through the ductwork, and most of the rest goes though the structural framework of the house, neither of which can be soundproofed very easily.

FURNACE RUNS TOO OFTEN?

The furnace in our home comes on a lot more frequently than the furnace in our last home. Right now, in cold weather, it comes on for six minutes and stays off for nine. I have had the furnace checked thoroughly and the thermostat replaced. The house temperature stays perfectly level; isn't it supposed to vary slightly?

Your furnace is cycling four times per hour, and there's nothing wrong with that. The frequency of the burner cycles depends on the size of the furnace, the outdoor temperature and the amount of insulation in your house, but about six times per hour is considered normal. The furnace will operate more efficiently, however, if the ON cycles are longer than this, which yours are.

The steady house temperature also indicates that your furnace and thermostat are working well. The temperature probably does fluctuate slightly, but this would be hardly noticeable on your new thermostat, which probably has Celsius markings.

FURNACE TURNS OFF TOO SOON

When our house thermostat turns the forced air furnace on, the fan starts about 30 seconds later, as it should, but before the room temperature gets up to the thermostat setting the burner shuts off again. The fan continues to run and the burner comes on again for about a minute. It can take six or seven cycles like this before the house gets up to temperature and the thermostat turns the burner off for a longer period. Then the whole routine starts again. Our furnace serviceman said the cold air duct was too small and cut another hole in it, but this didn't help at all.

There are only two things that can turn the burner off – the thermostat or the furnace safety control. The latter is a temperature sensing device that shuts the burner off if the temperataure inside the warm air plenum reaches the danger level, usually 200°F (93°C). A high temperature in the plenum could be caused by a very dirty filter that prevents the air from circulating through the plenum properly, but that should have been the first thing the serviceman checked. And I don't think *you* would have overlooked that. There could also be something wrong with the fan, and it is not moving as much air as it is supposed to. A loose fan belt could do that. It is also possible that the temperature limit setting on the safety control is set too low. The pointer on the fan control

dial cannot be set any *higher* than 200°F, but someone could easily have moved it lower by mistake.

A faulty thermostat could also be causing the burner to shut off too soon. The thermostat contains a device called an "anticipator" that turns the furnace off just *before* the room air reaches the temperature setting, allowing the heat that is still in the furnace to complete the job. An incorrect setting on the anticipator could cause it to turn the thermostat off too soon. If you remove the cover you will see a small numbered dial with a moveable pointer. Moving this to a higher number will make the furnace stay on longer. The furnace should only come on about six times an hour when the winter temperature is at its average level.

DISTRIBUTING HEAT FROM WOOD STOVE

My house is heated with a warm air gas furnace, but since I can get good firewood very cheaply I have installed a wood stove in the basement to reduce heating costs. Now the basement is very warm, particularly near the ceiling, and I would like to know how I can circulate this extra heat to the rest of the house.

If the cold air return duct going to the furnace passes over the wood stove or near it, all you have to do is cut a 3 ½ in. x 10 in. hole in the bottom or side of the duct, insert a grille, then use the manual switch on the furnace to turn the fan on and circulate the wood stove heat throughout the house via the existing duct system. If the cold air return duct is too far away, run a 5 in. branch duct over to the ceiling above the stove.

FLOOR SHIELD FOR WOOD STOVE

We have a Franklin wood stove in our cottage and would like to know what protection is needed for the wood floor, which is just 2 ft off the ground. Some people have suggested putting a layer of bricks under the stove. Will this do the job?

No. Although brick won't burn, it can conduct heat well enough to burn the floor underneath. The amount of protection that is needed depends on the construction of the stove, and should be explained in the manufacturer's literature. If such information is not available, the stove should be placed on a layer of hollow masonry blocks 4 in. thick. Below this you need a sheet of ¼ in. asbestos-cement board extending 18 in. in front of the stove and 6 in. on the other three sides and covered either with .022 in. sheet steel or ceramic tiles.

FLUE SIZE FOR WOOD STOVE

I have a small airtight wood stove in my basement, connected to a spare brick chimney. This is located on an outside wall and has a square tile flue lining. We are having trouble with creosote and black water running out of the chimney. What can we do to prevent this?

Allowing the fire to burn too slowly for too long is the main cause of this common problem. The relatively cool combustion gases containing water vapor and creosote condense inside the cold chimney.

Stovepipe thermometers that help you maintain the proper flue gas temperature to prevent condensation in the chimney are available at stores that sell wood stoves. But that masonry chimney will still be a problem. It's too big for the stove, for one thing. The size of the flue lining should match the size of the stovepipe. Your small stove probably takes a 5 in. stovepipe, and your chimney probably has an 8 in. x 8 in. flue tile. That's more that twice as large as it should be. (Even if you have 6 in. stovepipe, the flue tile is still 65% oversize.) The effect of this is to slow the passage of flue gases through the chimney, causing them to lose even more heat to the cold masonry.

If running your stove hotter doesn't cure the problem, the best remedy is to put a stainless steel liner in the chimney. This should be the same diameter as the stovepipe collar on the stove.

WOOD STOVE vs GAS FURNACE

I have been told that it is dangerous to use a wood stove in a basement with a gas furnace, but nobody can tell me why. The wood stove would not be in the same room as the furnace.

As long as enough outside air can get into the basement to supply the draft needs of both units going at the same time, there's no reason why you can't have a wood stove down there. But if the house is too well sealed the wood stove could draw air *down* the gas vent, bringing combustion gases back into the house. All you have to do is keep a nearby window open a bit.

RELINING A WOOD STOVE

We have a lovely old wood-burning range at our cottage. It works very well but the firebox is made of sheet metal lined with about half an inch of stove cement, and this only lasts two or three months. Is there some other way we can line the firebox?

You may be using the wrong type of lining. Ordinary stove cement is only made to fill cracks; it is not meant to be used as a lining material. For this, you need a special fireclay mixed with portland cement (3:1) and enough water to make a fairly stiff mortar. After it is applied to the firebox it should be kept damp for three days, then allowed to dry thoroughly before building a fire.

A better and faster job can be done with a product called Rutland Stove Lining #618. This is mixed with water, kneaded to a dough and pressed on the firebox walls. After one hour a small fire can be started in the stove; within a few hours it will take a full fire.

Sheet metal fireboxes are usually lined with firebricks, however, and you may be able to obtain the ones you need from the stove manufacturer. Regular firebricks are available as thin as 1 1/4 in. in a 9 in. x 4 1/2 in. size. It's best to use a "high duty" grade rated at 2500°F. You will also need a premixed refractory mortar. Both are available at stores that sell wood stoves and fireplace equipment.

SAFETY CLEARANCE FOR A WOOD STOVE

How much clearance should be allowed between a free-standing wood stove and a frame wall covered with gypsumboard and Z-Brick?

Both gypsumboard and Z-Brick are incombustible, but they conduct heat well enough to burn the wood frame wall behind them. Safety regulations call for a clearance of at least 36 in. between the stove and the wall.

The stove can be as close as 18 in. to the wall, however, if it is covered by a sheet of 1/4 in. asbestosboard faced with .013 in. sheet metal. Or as close as 12 in. if the asbestosboard is held 1 in. out from the wall on metal spacers. Prefabricated heat shields are available from the stores that sell wood stoves.

TWO STOVES ON ONE CHIMNEY

I have an outside brick chimney with a square tile lining. An airtight wood stove in my basement is connected to this and works very well. Now I would like to put a second airtight wood stove on the main floor. Can I connect this to the same chimney?

Section 21B.2 of the Residential Standards of the National Building Code, which is followed by most municipal and provincial building codes, specifically permits connecting two fuel-burning appliances (other than fireplaces) to one flue – provided they are on different levels and the flue is large enough to serve them both.

The standard 8x8 flue tile has an effective area only slightly less than two 6 in. stovepipes. Since it is extremely unlikely that you would ever have both stoves burning to capacity at the same time, you would seem to meet these requirements. Your local building department may have different ideas, however. Better check with them first.

HUMIDITY PROBLEMS

CEILING FAN DRIPS

We have an exhaust fan in the ceiling of the bathroom in our new home, and we're having a problem with it. If the fan is on while we're having a bath, water soon begins to drip out of it onto the floor. Sometimes it will drip even if the fan isn't on. Can you explain why this is happening and what we can do about it.

This is caused by the humid bathroom air condensing inside the cold vent pipe where it passes through the attic. The warm air will rise through this whether the fan is on or not. The remedy is to wrap the vent pipe in the attic with insulation batts, which can simply be tied on with string.

CONDENSATION IN ATTACHED GARAGE

We have an attached garage that can be entered directly from the kitchen. The garage is finished inside but unheated. Our problem is that the inside of the big garage door is covered with condensation during cold weather, and now mold is growing on the garage walls and ceiling. What is causing this? Would insulation help?

The problem is caused by warm, humid air leaking into the garage from the kitchen. Dampness due to condensation promotes the growth of mildew. Insulation would help, but it is difficult to insulate the finished wall, ceiling and door. What you can do, however, is weatherstrip the kitchen door to keep household air

from getting into the garage. You can also provide more ventilation in the garage to reduce the humidity there. This can be done by installing a couple of louvered vent openings in an outside wall.

CONDENSATION BEHIND BASEMENT WALLS

I insulated my basement last summer, putting tarpaper on the concrete walls first, then erecting 2x4 walls against them, putting R12 batts between the studs and finally covering the entire wall with polyethylene vapor barrier. When the cold weather came I noticed some water running out under the frame walls, and when I removed some of the insulation I found that it was wet and that water was running down the tarpaper behind it. Did I make a mistake in putting tarpaper on the foundation first?

No. This is recommended in the building code for the purpose of keeping the frame wall from coming into contact with the concrete below ground level, where dampness could lead to wood decay. The water running out under the wall is due to two things: too much humidity in your house, and an ineffective vapor barrier on the frame wall you put up. What is happening is that the humid household air is passing through or around your insulated wall and reaching the cold concrete (or the cold tarpaper on top of it), where it condenses, soaks the insulation and runs out under the bottom of the frame wall.

It is not enough just to staple sheets of polyfilm over the insulation. What you need is a completely airtight seal over the entire wall area. Overlapping sheets of vapor barrier must be sealed with tape or acoustic caulking compound. The plastic film should also extend up past the top of the frame wall and cover the batts you have (or should have) pushed between the ends of the joists. It must also be sealed to the sides of the joists and the floor above to prevent any air leakage there. Where two walls meet in a corner, the vapor barrier should be overlapped and sealed.

Such extreme precautions would not be necessary if you maintained a lower humidity level in your house (I suspect you are also having trouble with dripping windows) and this might be a lot easier to achieve now. If you have a humidifier on your furnace, the first thing to do is turn this off. If you do not use a humidifier, then the remedy is to provide more ventilation in the house to get rid of the moisture produced by cooking, washing, bathing, houseplants, etc. Opening windows or using an exhaust fan are simple ways to provide more ventilation. When your windows stop steaming up, you have the right amount of humidity. Keep the ventilation at that level and you should no longer have condensation behind your finished basement walls.

FURNACE CAUSES CONDENSATION

Last year I converted my forced warm air heating system from oil to gas, using a high efficiency, condensing type of furnace that has no chimney, just small intake and exhaust pipes that go directly outside. Now I am having trouble with heavy condensation and ice forming on the windows. Even some of the walls get damp and bedrooms are beginning to smell musty. The heating company told me to connect an outside air vent to the cold air return duct of the furnace, but this hasn't helped. Would it do any good to install a turbine ventilator in the roof, or use a dehumidifier?

The increased humidity in your house is due to the fact that you no longer have the ventilation provided by the former furnace and chimney, which drew a lot of outside air into the house. The new furnace has a closed combustion system that does not use household air. The advantage of this is that it reduces heat loss; the disadvantage is that it also reduces household ventilation, allowing the humidity produced by cooking, bathing, washing and even breathing, to build up to the point where condensation occurs on every cool surface.

The outside air duct will have done some good, but obviously not enough. The simple remedy for your problem – the *only* practical remedy, in fact – is to provide more ventilation. This can be done by installing an exhaust fan in the bathroom or kitchen (or both) where most of the humidity originates – or just by leaving a couple of windows open enough to stop the condensaiton forming on the windows. When this happens you will know you have enough ventilation; keep it more or less at that level. You will lose some heat by doing this, of course, but less, certainly,then you used to lose up the chimney, and the high efficiency furnace will still save you a lot of money.

A roof vent won't help the problem at all because it only ventilates the attic, not the house. And a dehumidifier won't work, either, because it can only take the humidity down to about 55% or 60%, which is fine in the summer but much too high to prevent condensation during the cold weather.

HUMIDIFIER vs SOFTENED WATER

I installed a drum-type humidifier on my furnace about two years ago, connecting it to the water line from our softener. It has always worked well but I read recently that softened water should not be used in humidifers. Why is that?

The calcium salts in hard water form a solid deposit when the water evaporates from the humidifier pad. A softener converts the calcium salts to soluable sodium salts, and these form a very fine, white powder on the humidifier pad that can be dispersed through the house by the furnace ductwork. You may not have realized that some of the dust on your furniture and other surfaces in the house was coming from your humidifier.

This can be eliminated by connecting the humidifer to an unsoftened water line. The pads will have to be replaced more often, or soaked periodically in an acid solution such as vinegar or one part muriatic acid to 20 parts water to remove the calcium deposits. You can also buy special conditioners that can be added to the water pan to prevent a buildup of hard deposits there.

KEROSENE HEATER CAUSES CONDENSATION

Ever since we started using a kerosene heater for auxiliary heat we have had a problem with heavy condensation and frost on our windows. What causes this? I would expect a heater to keep the air dry.

All hydrocarbons produce water vapor when they burn, and kerosene is no exception. With an unvented space heater like this, the water vapor stays in the house and raises the humidity level. In some homes the increased humidity is a benefit, but the level in your house must have been fairly high to start with, and the extra moisture has now raised it to the condensation point.

As with all condensation problems, the best remedy is to provide more ventilation to get rid of the humidity. When your windows no longer steam up you have the right amount of ventilaiton. Try to keep it at that level.

CONDENSATION ON STORM WINDOWS

We had storm windows installed last fall to conserve heat and stop condensation on the windows. Now we are getting condensation on the *storm* windows. What can we do to stop this?

Humid household air is now leaking past the inside windows and condensing on the cold outside pane. To prevent this, seal the joint between the inside window sash and the frame with weatherproofing tape or putty. Also check to make sure there is some ventilation behind the storm window. It should either fit a little loosely or have a few holes in the top and bottom of the frame to allow some outside air to circulate behind the glass.

CONDENSATION ON THERMAL WINDOWS

Two years ago I was getting some condensation on my living and dining room windows, which were fitted with old-fashioned storm windows. A salesman persuaded me to have the windows replaced with new ones that had sealed, double-glazed thermal units instead of storms. During the following fall and winter there was so much condensation on the windows that I had to keep towels on the sills to soak up the water, but some still ran down the walls and has ruined the plaster. The company that installed the windows now tells me this is normal, but that isn't what the salesman said. How can I correct this problem?

Sealed, double-glazed thermal window units are certainly better than single glazing, and they are more attractive and less trouble than storm windows. But consumers are rarely told that thermal units with an air space of less than half an inch between the panes actually provide less insulation than a properly fitted storm window. That means that your inside glass surface is colder than it was before, which is why you are getting more condensation.

The easiest remedy is to increase the ventilation in the house to lower the humidity. But adding a third pane, such as an outside storm window or a do-it-yourself plastic pane on the inside, will provide more insulation than you had originally, and should eliminate the condensation.

CONDENSATION ON TOILET TANK

During hot, humid weather, condensation forms on our toilet tank and drips constantly on the floor. I have heard that there is a paint of some kind that will stop this. Can you tell me what it is?

I know of no paint that will cure this problem, but there are two things you *can* do. The simplest is a plastic tray that hangs under the toilet tank to catch the drips. A neater remedy is to apply a layer of plastic foamboard insulation

about ¼ in. thick to the inside of the tank. This is available at most hardware stores in a kit that includes adhesive and instructions. (The job is not as easy as it sounds, however.) Both of these cost around $5.

DRIPPING WINDOWS

I have a moisture problem every year in my 30-year-old house. It takes two towels to soak up the puddles on my windowsills every morning. I have replaced the windows with double-glazed units that are much tighter than the old ones, weatherstripped the doors, added insulation to the attic, put on insulated aluminum siding, and added two roof vents. I also had an outside air duct connected to the furnace, but this let in a lot of cold air and didn't seem to be doing any good so I disconnected it. My neighbor's house is the same as mine but he never has this problem. I've been told my house is too airtight, but I'm sure newer houses are sealed much tighter than mine, and they don't seem to have this problem.

A great many new houses also have this problem, and for the same reason you do. Your house is too airtight *for the amount of humidity you produce.* This varies with each household, according to the number of occupants, amount and kind of cooking done, numbers of baths taken, etc., so you cannot compare one house with another. Ventilation is the only practical way to reduce humidity, unless you want to change your living habits. (A dehumidifier cannot get the humidity low enough to do the job in winter.)

Your added roof vents help to keep the attic free of condensation but they do nothing to ventilate the house. The other things you have done, such as replacing windows, weatherstripping doors and increasing insulation have saved heat, certainly, but they have also reduced the amount of ventilation in the house. This has allowed the humidity to build up until condensation forms on every cool surface, where it can cause considerabale damage to paint, insulation and the wood framework of your house. This damage will cost a lot more to repair than the modest amount you are saving in heat by not providing the ventilation that is needed.

To stop the condensation you must restore the ventilation you have lost. The first thing to do is reconnect the outside air duct to the furnace. You may also have to install an exhaust fan and keep it running *as long as the windows are steaming up.* (A better way to do this is to connect the exhaust fan to a humidistat that will turn it on whenever the humidity in the house gets too high.) It may be necessary to open a basement window close to the furnace, too, to be sure this is getting all the combustion air it needs.

EARLY CONDENSATION

The windows in my house only drip with condensation in the fall. When the really cold weather comes they stay dry. Why is this? I thought condensation was a winter problem.

A wet summer or fall adds moisture to everything in your house – carpets, linen, walls, floors, upholstered furniture, clothing, bedding, etc. When the first cool nights arrive, the indoor humidity is often still high enough to cause condensation to form on the cold windows. But after the heat has been on for a few weeks the house and its contents dry out and the condensation stops. Cold winter air is also much dryer than the warmer fall air when it is brought into the house by normal leakage and other ventilation, so this too keeps the indoor humidity down.

Unlike the more common winter condensation problems, early condensation like this can often be corrected by keeping a dehumidifier running in the house. (In colder weather the indoor humidity level required to prevent condensation is lower than a home dehumidifier can achieve.) You should also look for sources of household moisture that can be reduced, such as frequent shower baths (install an exhaust fan in the bathroom) or exposed soil in a crawlspace (cover with polyethylene film). And if you have a humidifier on your furnace, it should be turned off during the first few weeks of the heating season.

HEAT PUMPS AND HUMIDITY

About three years ago we replaced our oil furnace with an all-electric heat pump. Since then we have found the air in the house very stale most of the time. We are also getting a lot of condensation on the windows that we never had before. The people who installed the heating system say they have no idea what caused this. My son thinks we should connect an outside air duct to the cold air return duct of the furnace.

The problem is caused by lack of ventilation. Your oil furnace accounted for about 40% of all the ventilation you had in your house during the winter, because of the fresh air it drew in to maintain combustion and chimney draft. Electric heating brings in no fresh air at all, of course, because it has no chimney. To some extent this represents a heat saving, because you probably had more ventilation than you needed, but now you are not getting enough to remove the stale air and keep the humidity low enough to prevent condensation problems.

The remedy is very simple; just restore part of the ventilation you have lost. Your son's suggestion to install an outside air vent would work with a fuel-burning furnace but is not recommended with a heat pump because this only warms the air in the heating ducts to around 35°C (95°F), and a direct outside air intake would cool this below the comfort level.

Merely opening a couple of windows a bit for steady cross-ventilation will probably provide all the ventilation you need, but many people are reluctant to do this in cold weather, when the ventilation is needed most. A kitchen or bathroom exhaust fan may be more acceptable, but it is important to keep this running as long as condensation is forming on the windows.

HUMIDIFIER PRODUCES WHITE DUST

Since I started using an ultrasonic vaporizing humidifier I have been plagued with a deposit of fine white dust that settles on everything in the house. Where does this come from? Is there any way I can prevent it?

The dust consists of very fine particles of the hardness chemicals in your water supply (primarily calcium carbonate) that are left in the air when the water spray evaporates. The problem can only be corrected by using distilled water or a special demineralizing filter that should be available where you bought the humidifier. Water from a conventional softener will not help, incidentally, because this still contains dissoved mineral salts that will leave a white dust when the water evaporates.

HUMIDITY CONTROL FOR EXHAUST FAN

You have recommended adding a humidistat control to an exhaust fan so it would come on automatically to provide the ventilation needed when the indoor humidity gets too high. I have been unable to find such a control. Can you give me more information about it?

Two wall-mounted units are available. Honeywell model H46C can be obtained from any electrical or heating supply company. (If they don't have it in stock they can order it for you.) Leigh Metal Products, manufacturers of home ventilating equipment sold at most building supply stores, also have a humidistat, model 581, that can be used with an exhaust fan.

Technically, these are dehumidistats, since they turn on the fan when the humidity rises to a preset level. To control your exhaust fan you need one with a humidity range starting at 20%.

The setting you need will vary according to the outside temperature, and is best determined simply by watching your windows. When they begin to steam up, your house has all the humidity it can take; move the humidistat pointer down until the fan starts, then leave it at that setting for automatic operation. When the weather gets colder you may have to lower the setting; when it gets warmer you will be able to set the humidistat a little higher.

The humidistat should be wired in parallel with the manual on/off switch. If you don't know how to do this, call in an electrician.

INSULATION INCREASES HUMIDITY

In an effort to save energy we had the insulation in our attic increased from R8 to R36 last summer. But when the cold weather came the humidity level in our house soared, causing condensation not only on the windows but on the outside walls and baseboards. Mold has formed there, too, and we can smell the mildew in our clothes and bedding. This worries us particularly because we have a new baby in the house. What could be causing this and what can we do about it? Would a dehumidifier help?

The new baby has more to do with the problem than the insulation, I think. The extra cooking, bathing, washing and drying have increased the humidity in your house to the point where condensation forms when the air is even slightly cooled. Ordinary household dehumidifiers can only take the humidity down to about 60%, and that is still much too high to prevent condensation and mildew in cold weather. You would need an industrial dehumidifier, and this is neither economical nor practical for residential use.

There's a much simpler remedy in any case. All you need is ventilation to replace some of the humid air with relatively dry outside air. An exhaust fan in the bathroom – and perhaps the kitchen, too – would certainly help, but just keeping a couple of windows open a bit will do the job. If you have a warm air heating system, you can have an outside air duct connected directly to the cold air return duct. In this way the air will be heated and filtered before it circulates through the house. For about $50 you can buy a unit with a thermostatically-controlled damper that prevents air being drawn into the house unless the heat is on.

The increased insulation will have contributed to the problem slightly, however, because it reduced air leakage through the ceiling. Usually this is a good thing, but in your case you need all the ventilation you can get. The added insulation also reduced the amount of time your furnace is on, and this, too, decreased the amount of fresh air being brought into the house.

HUMIDITY vs TEMPERATURE

The instructions on our power humidifier say that we must reduce the indoor humidity when the outside temperature decreases. They recommend a humidity setting of 35% when the temperature is -7°C (19°F), and a humidity level of only 15% when the temperature is -29°C (-30°F). Why is this?

When the outside temperature drops, a lower indoor humidity is necessary in order to prevent condensation on the cold windows and walls. The "dew point" depends on two factors: the amount of humidity in the air and the temperature of the surface. Even though the air temperature in the house is kept fairly constant, the windows, walls and even the perimeter of an insulated ceiling will be cooled by the loss of heat as the temperature outside drops, and condensation will form on them if the humidity is high enough. The lower the outside temperature, the less humidity you can have in the house. It's really very simple once you realize what is happening.

HUMIDIFIER NECESSARY?

The air in our house has always been very dry and we were thinking of installing a humidifier. Which type is best, a portable unit or a central one on the furnace?

They will both do the same job, but a furnace humidifier requires less attention. Either one is an expensive way to increase the humidity in your home, however. It takes nearly 10,000 BTU of heat energy to vaporize one gallon of water, no matter what kind of humidifier you use. In very cold weather you may need several gallons, which would be equivalent to running your furnace for about half an hour.

There is a much cheaper way to do it. *The only reason the air in your house is dry during cold weather is because you have too much air leakage.* Cold outside air becomes very dry when it is warmed to house temperature, and this is what causes the indoor humidity to drop.

Normal household activities such as cooking, bathing, washing, watering house plants, etc, produce enough moisture to keep the indoor humidity at a comfortable level *if you don't have too much air leakage.* Reducing the air leakage by caulking and weatherstripping will not only increase the humidity in your home during the winter months, it will also reduce your heating costs.

But if you reduce the air leakage too much the humidity will go too high and you will start getting condensation problems. Start by weatherstripping the doors and windows that are particularly drafty, then wait a few days and watch the windows for signs of condensation. If there are none, continue to seal other leaks, but as soon as you see the windows beginning to steam up you will know that the house has the right level of ventilation. This is the only practical way to judge the humidity/ventilation level in your home.

HUMIDIFIER IN ELECTRIC FURNACE

I have installed a new 20-kilowatt electric warm air furnace in place of my old oil furnace. A drum-type humidifier was connected between the cold air return plenum and the warm air plenum on the old furnace. Can I install it in the new furnace the same way?

The only thing to watch is that you don't put the humidifier where water could drip on the electric heating elements. Normally it is located on the return air side with a bypass duct to the warm air plenum.

But I don't think you shoulld install a humidifier at all until you have seen what the humidity level is in your house next winter. Switching from a fuel-burning furnace to an electric furnace will raise the humidity anyway, because it eliminates the ventilation provided by the chimney. In other words, it doesn't bring in as much cold and relatively dry outside air. This reduced ventilation saves heat, of course, but it can also cause serious condensation problems. You may find you need to provide more ventilation to keep the humidity *down* next winter.

HUMIDIFIER TAKES HEAT

Our gas furnace has a drum type humidifier installed on the warm air plenum. A duct runs from this to the cold air return plenum. I have always been under the impression that any leakage from the warm air side of the furnace to the cold air side would reduce its efficiency. Isn't this method of installation just wasting heat?

The bypass system for exterior-mounted humidifiers does not, in itself, reduce the heat output of the warm air furnace. It merely recirculates some of the warm air through the humidifier and back into the return duct. This small detour does not reduce the efficiency of the furnace.

What does reduce the heat output, however, is the evaporation of the water in the humidifier. This lowers the temperature of the air significantly. It takes 10,000 BTUs of heat to evaporate a gallon of water, and many homes require four gallons or more a day to maintain household humidity at the desired level during very cold weather. The average furnace must burn for nearly half an hour to produce this much heat.

Any other method of adding moisture to the air – such as a vaporizer or portable humidifier – will require just as much energy, however. There *is* a way to increase the humidity and lower fuel consumptionm, however. Reduce air leakage by caulking and weatherstripping.

WHERE DOES FURNACE HUMIDISTAT GO?

Our house has a natural gas furnace with a drum-type humidifier located on the cold air return side of the furnace. A four-inch flexible pipe connects it to the main warm air supply plenum. The humidistat (humidity sensor) that operates the drum motor is also located on the warm air supply plenum. Someone has told me this should be on the cold air return side, and I was wondering if this could be the reason why we are having a problem with condensation on our windows.

The humidifier itself is properly installed, but the humidistat should not be located on the output side of the furnace. The warm air here is a lot drier than the air on the return side, so the humidifier will be running when it is not needed. The humidistat should be located on the cold air return side of the furnace, where it will be measuring the humidity level of the air coming from every room in the house, and this is as close to a true average figure as you can get.

VAPORIZER IN BABY'S ROOM

There is a heavy growth of mildew on the plaster walls and ceiling of our baby's room, where we are using a vaporizer to maintain a healthy humidity. The dripping windows are also causing the paint on the sills to crack. Is there a remedy to our problem?

The problem is due to excessive humidity in this room, of course. The mildew can be removed with a strong solution of chlorine laundry bleach - one part to four parts water - but this and other problems caused by condensation will keep coming back if you continue to use the vaporizer. Your house was not built to take this much moisture and there is no way to adapt it to such use now. It is questionable if a humidity level this high is desirable, in any case. Hospital nurseries are not kept anywhere near as humid as this. Check with your doctor; he will probably recommend less humidity and more fresh air.

DEHUMIDIFIER DOES NOT WORK

We have had a lot of trouble with condensation during the winter – dripping windows, mold on the walls, mildew in the closets – so this year I bought a dehumidifier to get rid of it. Although it is an expensive model that is suppose to extract three gallons of water a day, I only get a couple of quarts out of it and the windows are still dripping.

A dehumidifier can only reduce the humidity to about 60%, which is a great improvement on a hot summer day when the humidity may be 80% or 90%, but it is much too high to prevent condensation problems in winter, when walls and windows are much cooler. So although it may seem like a logical thing to do, using a dehumidifier is not a remedy for *winter* condensation problems. The only practical remedy for that is increased ventilation to get rid of the moisture produced by such normal household activities as cooking, bathing, washing and watering houseplants.

DEHUMIDIFIER ICES UP

The dehumidifier we use in our basement has worked fine for several years, but this summer the coils are getting covered with ice and then the dehumidifier shuts off. What would cause this?

There are several possible causes. Perhaps the air temperature in your basement is unusually low this year. If the humidity is high and the temperature drops below 18°C (65°F), the evaporator coils that draw the moisture out of the air can get cold enough to turn the condensation to frost. Some frosting is normal for a few minutes after the dehumidifier starts, but if it continues to build up the safety control will turn the compressor off.

Anything that reduces the flow of air through the dehumidifier can also cause it to ice up. Perhaps the fan isn't working properly, or the fins on the condenser unit behind the cold evaporator coils may be clogged with dust. Even placing the dehumidifier too close to a wall can reduce the flow of air through the unit.

USING A DEHUMIDIFIER UPSTAIRS

We use a dehumidifier in the basement of our bungalow during the summer. We were thinkng of buying another one to use upstairs but the salesman told us that a dehumidifier will only work in the basement. I'm sure he was being honest because he lost a sale with this advice, but I'm still not convinced he's right.

He may be honest, but he's wrong – or partly wrong in any case. A dehumidifier will remove just as much moisture from humid air upstairs as it will in the basement. But extracting the water does produce a lot of heat, and this can make the closed rooms upstairs uncomfortably warm. Basements are usually cooler, so the heat from the dehumidifier is not so noticeable.

A window air conditioner would probably be a better investment because it cools *and* dehumidifies. Your honest salesman may be rewarded with a good sale after all.

INSULATION

ATTIC INSULATION COOLS BASEMENT

We had 12 in. of insulation put in the ceiling of our one-storey home last fall. Our problem is that this has made the uninsulated basement very cold. It never used to be before we insulated the attic. How could this have caused the basement to get cold, and what can we do about it?

This sounds very strange, but actually there's a fairly simple explanation. The insulation in the attic has kept the living area much warmer, so the thermostat here does not turn the furnace on as often as it used to. And since much of the heat in the basement comes from the furnace itself, this has allowed the basement to get colder. The remedy is to insulate the basement walls, which will reduce your heating costs even more.

INSULATING AN A-FRAME COTTAGE

I would like to know how to insulate the sloping walls of an A-frame cottage. The walls are shingled over plywood sheathing, and the 2x6 rafters are exposed inside. I was thinking of gluing 2 in. polystyrene foam-

board to the sheathing between the rafters and covering this with gypsumboard to leave 3 in. of the rafters still exposed. Will this work?

Any insulation is better than none, but 2 in. of foamboard will only give you an added insulation value of R8 to R10. You should have at least R20. The most practical way to do this is to put 6 in., R20 fibreglass batts between the rafters, cover them with a vapor barrier of polyethylene film, then apply wall panelling. To maintain the exposed beam effect, nail 2x3 (on edge) through the panelling to the hidden rafters.

INSULATING BALLOON FRAME WALLS

We have an old 2-storey house with balloon frame walls that contain no insulation. How can we insulate them?

In modern frame construction, wall studs only span the distance from one floor platform to the next. In balloon frame construction, the studs extend from the foundation to the attic. (The floor joists are supported on a ledger board nailed to the studs.)

This means there is a 2-storey wall cavity between the studs, which can be filled with insulation blown through holes drilled in the top of the wall from the attic. Cross-bracing and windows will block some areas, however, so it takes an experienced and conscientious applicator to do the job properly. Cellulose fibre insulation is easiest to apply and gives the best R value in this situation.

BASEMENT INSULATION

The joists in our basement ceiling are recessed into the poured concrete foundation wall, with only 2 or 3 in. projecting above it. When I was insulating the basement I was told to push batts between the ends of the joists, but we live in a very cold area and this has made the perimeter of the floor upstairs very cold. Should I take the insulation out or leave it there?

Although still practiced in some areas, this is now an uncommon method of connecting the floor joists to the foundation walls. Usually the joists rest on 2x4 or 2x6 sill plates bolted to the top of the foundation wall. Since such joists are entirely above the foundation, it is correct to put insulation between them. But when the joists are partly embedded in the foundation wall, as yours are, there is a gap of only a few inches between the top of the wall and the floor above. Stuffing this with insulation will keep the heat of the basement from warming the perimeter of the floor above, and in very cold areas like yours the wall-floor joint in these rooms can get cold enough for frost to form on the baseboards.

The government handbook on home insulation, *Keeping The Heat In*, recommends leaving a 1-in. space between the insulation and the floor, but I would leave the insulation out of this space entirely.

INSULATING BASEMENT WALLS

I want to insulate my basement, but can't decide which of two methods to use. One is to strap the walls with 2x4s every 16 in. and put in 4 in. batt insulation, then apply a vapor barrier and panelling. The other is to strap the walls with 2x2s every 48 in. and put 2 in. of white foamboard insulation between them, covering this with gypsumboard. Which method would provide the most insulation at the best price?

It isn't practical to strap the walls with 2x4s on edge; you could never nail them to the concrete that way. The way to use 2x4s is to build a free standing frame wall with them – vertical studs between top and bottom plates against the concrete wall. Then you can put in 3½ in., R12 batts and cover them with vapor barrier and the panelling of your choice. The studs should be spaced 24 in. on centres and filled with 23½ in. wide batts.

Your 2x2 strapping is only 1½ in. thick (as the 2x4s are only 3½ in.) and this much foamboard has an insulation value of around R6, only half the R value of the batts. You would have to use 3 in. foamboard to achieve the same insulation value, and the wall would cost more than conventional frame construction with batts.

INSULATING ABOVE BASEMENT WALL

I have insulated my basement walls up to the ceiling joists, using 2x4 framing, R12 batt insulation and polyethylene vapor barrier. Should I also put insulation between the ends of the joists? And if so, how can I cover this with an airtight vapor barrier?

Normally there is no insulation at all around the outside of the floor platform that sits on the foundation walls, so a lot of heat can be lost there. Insulation should be placed not only between the *ends* of the joists that rest on the two side walls of the foundation, but also on the *sides* of the joists that lie on the two end walls. You should insulate the entire perimeter of the floor platform, in other words, not just two sides.

Fibreglass or mineral wool batt insulation is difficult to install and cover with a vapor barrier in these areas, so I recommend using polystyrene foamboard – at least 2 in. thick. The common white foamboard will do. This can be glued in place by applying a bead of panel adhesive around the back edge of the foamboard and then pressing it in place. No vapor barrier is necessary because the foamboard itself is reasonably impervious to moisture vapor.

INSULATING A CATHEDRAL CEILING

Our house was built in 1965 and has a large cathedral ceiling in the main living area. The ceiling consists of tongue-and-groove cedar planking on exposed beams spaced 48 in. apart. We don't think there is much insulation up there, and would like to increase it.

I doubt that you will have more than an inch of fibreboard insulation on top of the plank ceiling, and the total R value is probably less than 6. You're loosing a lot of heat up there, but you have only two places you can insulate a cathedral ceiling – either inside or outside. Outside is best because it doesn't change the look of the ceiling, but insulating inside can be cheaper.

If you happen to need a new roof, anyway, it would be best to have the insulation applied at the same time. The old shingles should be removed and 4 in. of foamboard insulation applied. The common white foamboard is satisfactory and relatively inexpensive, but urethane foamboard has the highest insulation value. One-by-three strapping should be nailed through this into the plank deck and then covered with plywood or chipboard sheathing. (The purpose of the strapping is to provide some ventilation under the sheathing to keep the shingles from getting too hot during the summer.) Shingles can then be applied to the sheathing.

If you prefer to insulate the ceiling from the inside, glue at least 2 in. of foamboard to the plank decking between the beams, then cover it with gypsumboard panels nailed through to the decking or held in place with strips of molding nailed to the beams. The gypsumboard can be painted, of course, but plywood or lumber can be used instead if you want to preserve the appearance of the wood ceiling.

INSULATING A COLD STORAGE ROOM

I am converting a small cold cellar under our front porch to a basement clothes closet. I put 1x2 strapping on the concrete walls and ceiling and applied 2 in. foamboard insulation over this. When I removed

a piece of the foamboard to install a lighting fixture I discovered that the concrete behind it was very wet. Should I apply some kind of waterproofing material to the concrete?

No. The moisture is due to condensation from humid household air that is able to get behind the foamboard because you have put it on top of the strapping. The foamboard should be glued directly to the concrete. Another way to do this is to nail 2x2 strapping to the concrete and glue 1½ in. of foamboard (the thickness of the 2x2s) to the concrete between the strapping, then screw or nail gypsumboard to the strapping. In either case, be sure to use an adhesive that is compatible with the polystyrene foamboard. Apply a bead of adhesive around the back of the foamboard, about an inch from the edge; this will keep humid air from getting behind the insulation and condensing on the cold concrete.

Another way to do this job is to use a special type of foamboard that is grooved to take 1x2 wood or metal strapping. Holes are drilled through the strapping and foamboard into the concrete to take special nails. Most building supply stores carry these materials or can get them for you.

INSULATING COTTAGE FLOOR

I have a holiday cottage located on a lake. The flooring is ¾ in. plywood covered with resilient tile. The crawlspace under the floor is open and high enough to work in. I plan to insulate the floor with R20 batts pushed up between the joists and covered with ¼ in. plywood. Do I need a vapor barrier to prevent condensation in the insulation, and if so, where does it go?

If you keep the humidity in the cottage low enough during cold weather to prevent the windows from dripping, it is unlikely that you will need a vapor barrier between the floor and the insulation. But if you want to be on the safe side, either use batts with a vapor barrier face or cut strips of 4-mil polyethylene film 30 in. wide and wrap them over the top and sides of the batts before you push them up between the joists. Until the sheathing is applied, the batts can be held there with 15 in. lengths of coathanger wire wedged between the joists. Since ventilation underneath the insulation is desirable, perforated hardboard would make better sheathing than plywood. Quarter-inch wire screen, or "hardware cloth", could also be used. Either of these will let the air in but keep vermin out.

INSULATING A METAL CHIMNEY

A couple of years ago I installed an insulated metal chimney on the outside of my house to serve an airtight stove in my basement rumpus room. This works fine as long as there is a brisk fire in the stove, but when the fire is low and the weather is very cold, the chimney doesn't draw properly and smoke comes into the room. Would it help if I put fibreglass insulation around the chimney and boxed it in?

Adding insulation like this could cause the chimney to overheat, and is not approved by Underwriters' Laboratories of Canada (ULC), the main testing authority for this product. I don't think it's necessary, in any case. It would be enough to box in the chimney to shelter it from wind and provide a little insulation, leaving a 2 in. air space around the chimney.

Check, too, to make sure you have enough ventilation in the basement to maintain the chimney draft. Try opening a nearby window a bit when the stove begins to smoke. There's a good chance that this will solve the problem.

INSULATING CRAWLSPACE

A couple of years ago I put a new forced air heating system in my house. There is a basement under the front of the house, but two bedrooms at the back are over a crawlspace. The heating ducts to these rooms pass through the crawlspace, and I think they should be insulated to conserve heat. "Not so," says the contractor, who claims the heat will keep the floors of the rooms above warm. What is your advice?

The contractor is right, but he should have suggested insulating the walls of the crawlspace in order to conserve heat. Glue sheets of polystyrene foamboard or rigid fibreglass, at least 2 in. thick, directly to the inside of the foundation walls, hang insulation batts down the foundation walls after fastening them to the header between the joists. If there is an earth floor in the crawlspace, it should be covered with 6-mil polyethylene film to keep down the humidity. This can be held in place with stones or a few shovelsful of gravel.

INSULATING OLD FARMHOUSE

I have a 100-year-old, 1½-storey stone farmhouse that I want to remodel and use as a year-round recreational home. We will only have the main floor finished at first, so I plan to put insulation in the ceiling here and close in the stairwell. I would like to know how to insulate the upstairs rooms and what to do about ventilating the attic.

Insulating the main floor ceiling before you get around to finishing the upstairs rooms isn't a very good idea, since the insulation will ultimately be wasted. The only way it will save any heat when the upstairs rooms are finished is by keeping them too cold. It would be much better to rough in the attic rooms now and insulate them in the usual way. Panelling and other finishing work can be left until later, however.

Put batt or loose fill insulation between and over the floor joists in the small attic spaces outside the short knee walls in the upstairs rooms. Strips of polyethylene vapor barrier 20 in. wide should be placed in the joist spaces before the insulation is applied. Place batts between the studs in the knee walls and between the rafters in what will be the sloping wall of the attic rooms. Insulation should also be placed above the small upstairs ceiling. Walls and ceiling should be covered with vapor barrier film before the panelling is applied.

The three attic spaces (outside the knee walls and above the small ceiling) should be ventilated as well as possible. The old house probably has a relatively airtight attic with no ventilation under the eaves, so you will have to use gable vents or roof vents, depending on the construction of the house.

INSULATING FRAME WALLS

The ceiling of our bungalow is insulated, but we have no insulation at all in the frame walls. Because there is stucco on the outside, I think it would be cheaper to apply insulation to the inside wall, and I plan to use 2 in. of polyethylene foamboard. This will be covered with gypsumboard and then painted. Is this the correct way to do it?

The best way to insulate your walls is to have cellulose fibre or fibreglass wool blown into the wall cavity. This can be done from the inside or outside, and the holes patched. Ask several contractors for bids and advice on whether inside or outside application would be best in your case.

This will give you about R12 in added insulation, or a total of around R15 for the wall, and will reduce heat loss there by about 80%. Since you are probably loosing about 40% of your heat through the walls now, the added insulation could reduce your heating bill by as much as one-third. You could add more insulation by applying rigid foamboard to the inside wall, as you suggest, but the cost is not justified by the small reduction in heating costs - perhaps another 5%, at best.

INSULATING GARAGE/HOUSE WALL

A concrete block wall separates our house from the attached garage. The wall is finished on the inside of the house but is not insulated, and I would like to apply some insulation from the garage side without taking up too much space. What do you recommend?

You can put up a standard 2x4 stud wall with batt insulation and panelling, but an easier way to do it is to apply rigid insulation panels directly to the masonry walls. I would use the 4 ft x 8 ft rigid fibreglass panels made for insulating the outside of basement walls. These are only 2 in. thick but have an insulation value of R8.5, or about three times as much as the existing wall. The fibreglass panels can be applied to the masonry wall with any of the construction or panel adhesives. If you want to cover the fibreglass surface with something to improve the appearance of the garage, I suggest brushing it with a white, washable, fire resistant coating such as Flintguard 120-18, made by Bakelite and available through building supply dealers.

INSULATING MASONRY WALLS

Our house is built of concrete block with stucco outside and gypsumboard on wood strapping inside. There is no insulation in the walls. The ¾ in. space behind the gypsumboard is too small to have insulation blown in, I'm told, so I have started cutting slots in the panelling and inserting strips of ½ in. thick foamboard in this empty space. This makes the wall noticeably warmer, but it's a very slow, messy job. Is there some covering like cork or panelboard that could be applied to the inside wall without taking up too much space?

As built, your walls have an insulation value of R2.6, which is very poor. Half an inch of the common white foamboard adds about R2. This will reduce the heat loss by around 40%, but it will still be very high – about the same as an uninsulated wood frame wall.

There are no thin wallcoverings that will provide any significant amount of insulation. Cork has about the same insulation value as foamboard and is a lot more expensive. Even urethane foamboard, the best of the common insulation materials, is only about one-third better (R6 per inch instead of R4).

It wouldn't take up much room to add 2 in. of the common foamboard and a layer of gypsumboard to the inside walls. Both can be applied with panel adhesive, and no vapor barrier is required. This will give the walls a total insulation value of around R10 and cut the heat loss by 75%.

In some cases, however, it may be easier or more desirable to apply insulation to the *outside* of the walls and then cover it with siding. Vertical 2x2 strapping must be applied to the wall first with a nailing gun, and foamboard insulation glued between the strapping (1½ in. will be the maximum thickness of insulation you have room for) before the siding is applied. Although it provides an attractive exterior finish, the siding itself will not add any notable amount of insulation.

INSULATING A METAL DOOR

The metal door that leads from our laundry room to the attached, unheated garage apparently doesn't contain any insulation, because it's very cold. How can I insulate it?

The ½ in. thick softboard or fibreglass panels used in suspended ceilings will provide a reasonable amount of insulation when applied to both sides of the door with panel adhesive.

INSULATING PLASTER WALLS

Our house was built in the '40s, and the basement has been finished with plaster walls and ceiling. There is no insulation in the walls, and we would like to know how we can add some without having to remove all the plaster.

You can glue the common white foamboard insulation directly to the plaster, using a construction adhesive that is compatible with polystyrene, then cover this with gypsumboard applied the same way. You should use at least 2 in. of foamboard. Plywood or hardboard can be used in place of gypsumboard, if preferred.

ROOF INSULATION

We have an old house with a large attic that is just used for storage. There is insulation only between the floor joists at present. Would it help if we placed additional insulation batts between the roof rafters?

No. The attic should be ventilated to the outside, so putting insulation under the roof would do no good. Simply add more insulation between the floor joists, or on top of them. It may be necessary to provide a raised floor for the items that are stored there. This can be done by toenailing 2x4s or 2x6s at right angles to the existing joists.

INSULATING A FLAT ROOF

We have a peaked roof over the front section of our house and a flat tar-and-gravel roof over the back half. We have insulated the attic in the peaked section but can't figure out how to put insulation between the roof joists in the flat roof. Can you tell me the best way to insulate this?

This type of roof is usually insulated by blowing cellulose fibre or fibreglass into the roof cavity, either by removing the fascia board at the ends of the joists or by cutting holes in the roof. But there are many reports of problems with this method caused by condensation forming on the underside of the roof sheathing, often leading to serious wood decay.

Research by a renovation company indicates that the remedy is to add 4 in. of foamboard insulation on top of the roof as well. One way to do this is to rake the gravel back, lay the foamboard on the roof, and then cover it with the gravel, adding more if necessary, to hold it in place. But if the present roof membrane is in poor condition, it is better to apply a new 4-ply roof and apply the foamboard to this before the gravel is put on.

This provides a total insulation value of at least R40 in the roof, and the added layer of foamboard virtually eliminates the possibility of condensation within the roof cavity. It's not a cheap solution, however.

INSULATING A MANSARD ROOF

I would like to put more insulation in the upstairs wall of our house, which has a mansard-style roof. How can I get insulation behind the sloping roof sections outside these walls?

There isn't much space to work in, but it can be done. If you remove the soffit panels under the overhang you will see that insulation can be applied directly to the sheathing panels on the outside of the house walls, between the mansard roof supports. This can be done by using at least 2 in. of rigid insulation such as polystyrene foamboard or the fibreglass panels made for insulating foundation walls (both are available at any building supply store). Cut the insulation to fit between the roof supports, apply dabs or beads of construction adhesive to the back of the insulation, then push it up inside the mansard roof and press it against the sheathing. One nail at the bottom will hold each insulation panel in place until the adhesive sets.

INSULATING SLAB FLOOR

We live in a one-storey, wood frame, basementless house with a concrete slab floor. Is there any way we can put insulation under the floor so that it won't be so cold next winter?

That would be very difficult, and it's unnecessary, anyway. Very little heat is lost to the earth below the slab; most of the heat loss is around the outside edges. This can be prevented by digging down 2 ft and applying 4 in. foamboard to the edge of the slab and its foundation. Any foamboard exposed above the ground should be covered with a packaged exterior stucco mix. Joints should be sealed first with self-adhesive fibreglass drywall joint tape. And the top edge of the insulation should be covered with a metal flashing strip tucked up under the siding. For added protection, paint the stucco with an exterior latex.

ASBESTOS INSULATION

We have a warm air heating system and some years ago we insulated the exposed ductwork in the basement with asbestos paper. Could loose fibres from this be blowing around the house and endangering our health?

There's a chance of that, certainly. Asbestos paper does not provide much insulation, in any case; fibreglass batts would do a much better job. But removing the asbestos paper would expose you to more fibres than just leaving it where it is. I would simply wrap fibreglass insulation over the asbestos and tie it in place with string.

ASBESTOS INSULATION ON PIPES

We have a hot water heating system in our house, and all the pipes exposed in the basement are covered with asbestos insulation. I understand this is a health hazard. How can we remove it, and will this increase our heating bills?

The main purpose of the insulation on the pipes is to reduce the amount of heat radiated into the basement. Removing it would still keep the heat in the house but would not distribute it as efficiently. The operation of taking the asbestos off the pipes would create more of a hazard than leaving it on. The simplest thing to do is wrap the asbestos with 2 in. wide plastic packaging tape, available at any stationary store. This will prevent asbestos fibres from getting into the air.

ATTIC INSULATION MAKES BASEMENT COLD

We had 12 in. of insulation put in the ceiling of our 1-storey home last fall. Our problem is that this has made our basement very cold. It never used to be before we insulated the attic. How could attic insulation have caused this, and what can we do about it?

This sounds ridiculous, but actually there's a fairly simple explanation. The thermostat for your heating system is on the main floor. The insulation in the ceiling has kept the living area much warmer, so the furnace doesn't come on as often as before, and this allows your uninsulated basement to get colder. The remedy is to insulate the basement walls, which will save even more heat.

COLD BEDROOM OVER GARAGE–1

One of our bedrooms is located over the garage and we can't seem to get it warm. There is R32 insulation in the ceiling, R12 in the walls and R20 in the floor. There is only one window and it is double-glazed and well sealed. The warm air heating system keeps the rest of the house at a comfortable temperature. Why would this one room be cold?

There are several possibilities. The heating duct to that room must pass over the garage ceiling, and it may not be insulated very well. The room is probably a long way from the furnace, and the duct system may not have been balanced (by adjusting dampers in the ducts) to get the required amount of warm air going to this room. The ducts leading to the other rooms should be closed a bit, in other words, to force more heat into this cold bedroom. Another possibility is the lack of a cold air return grille close to this room; you can't force warm air into it if there isn't some way for the cooled air to get back to the furnace. And finally, there may be some air leakage from the unheated garage into the floor cavity under the bedroom.

COLD BEDROOM OVER GARAGE–2

Our master bedroom is over the garage and the floor is very cold, even though it is carpeted and the ceiling of the garage has been covered with 2 in. of foamboard insulation.

If that's all the insulation you have in the bedroom floor, there are three things wrong with it. 1) It only has a value of R8 or R10 (depending on whether it's white or blue), and you need at least twice that. 2) If cold air is blowing through the ceiling cavity, which it probably is, insulation underneath the ceiling isn't doing much good, anyway. 3) Polystyrene foamboard is a fire hazard and should not be left exposed in a garage. It should be covered with gypsumboard. My advice is to have the ceiling cavity filled with cellulose fibre or fibreglass blowing wool insulation before the gypsumboard is applied.

BEDROOM FLOOR COLD

We have a split-level house in which two of the upstairs bedrooms overhang the lower floor by about 3 ft. During the winter, these rooms are much colder than the rest of the house, and you can feel the cold floor above the overhang even through the carpeting. What can we do to correct this?

Remove the soffit panelling under the overhang to see what insulation, if any, is under the floor. More can be added by pushing friction fit batts up between the floor joists. You should have at least 6 in. of batt insulation.

INSULATION BLOCKS SOFFIT VENTS

I had 12 in. of insulation blown into my attic last fall, and I think the workmen who did it have blocked all the ventilation openings into the attic from the roof overhang. How can I pull the insulation back from the rafters without having to walk on a sea of insulation and perhaps put my foot through the ceiling? I have no idea where the joists are.

You don't have to go into the attic to clear the insulation away from the rafters where they pass over the outside walls. This area can be reached from outside by removing the soffit panelling under the overhang. You can either push the loose insulation back into the attic or slip cardboard or plastic vent chutes between the insulation and the roof. These are available at most building supply stores.

CARPET AS INSULATION

Our master bedroom is directly over an unheated garage, and this makes the floor very cold. What type of carpet would provide the most insulation?

The thickness of the carpet is the most important factor, but 1¼ in. (32mm) is about as thick as you can get. There is not much difference in the insulation value of the different carpet fibres, according to studies done for the Canadian Carpet Institute, but wool does rate the highest, followed closely by polyester, nylon, acrylic and polypropylene, in that order. With any fibre, the insulation value also increases with the density of the pile, which generally increases with price.

There is a bigger difference in the insulation value of underpad materials. The relatively cheap urethane foams provide nearly twice as much insulation as the foam or sponge rubber underpads, but they are not considered as comfortable to walk on. For the warmest floor, then, you should put down ½ in. (13mm) urethane underpad (R2 in insulation value) and the thickest wool carpet you can afford (R2.6 per inch). At best, however, this will only give you R5.6 in added floor insulation. You can get more than R20 by blowing insulation into the garage ceiling or putting fibreglass batts between the joists.

COLD KITCHEN FLOOR

There seems to be something wrong with the insulation in the kitchen of our new home. The vinyl floor is very cold for 2 or 3 ft out from the cupboards. The kitchen is over the laundry room in the basement, where the ceiling is unfinished but the room is warm and there is no sign of a draft. Why is our kitchen floor so cold and how can we correct it?

The problem is caused by cold air coming into or under the cupboards, then spilling out over the kitchen floor. There are a number of devious routes the outside air can take, and most of them are easy to seal when the house is being built but difficult to do afterwards. Unfortunately our building codes do not yet require all of these well-known leakage points to be sealed, but some of the better builders do it anyway. Before buying a new home you should ask the builder to show you extra steps he has taken to seal these areas.

The hole where the drain pipe enters the wall under the sink is one place where cold air can enter. The gap is often hidden by a loose-fitting cover or flange, but it can still let a lot of cold air into the cupboard under the sink. Cold air can also get into the space between the kitchen floor and the bottom shelf of the cupboards, then spill out over the floor through gaps above and below the recessed kick strip. If your kitchen happens to overhang the foundation wall, which is not uncommon in split-level houses, then the air may be leaking in around the edge of the subfloor inside the overhang. Lack of insulation here would contribute to the problem.

It is very difficult to locate and seal all such leaks, however, and in many cases the simplest remedy is to remove the kick strip under the cupboards and use a piece of wood to push fibreglass batting to the back of the space under the cupboards, packing it tightly to block air leakage into the kitchen.

PROTECTING FOAMBOARD INSULATION

We were planning to apply foamboard insulation to the concrete walls of our unfinished basement, but have been told that this is a fire hazard and must be protected with a fireproof coating of some kind. Is this true?

Although all polystyrene foamboard insulation contains a fire retardant and will not support a flame (take the flame away and the fire goes out, in other words), it certainly does burn rapidly in a fire and also produces very toxic fumes. Building codes require that all foamboard insulation be protected with a fire barrier. Gypsumboard is preferred because of its high fire rating, but plywood, hardwood and particleboard are acceptable. Check your building department for any special requirements.

INSULATION INCREASES HUMIDITY

Two years ago I had R40 insulation blown into my attic. Ever since then there has been an excessive amount of condensation on our windows and even some mildew on the walls. What causes this and what can I do about it?

Too much humidity is the basic cause. The added insulation contributed to this in two ways: it reduced air leakage through the ceiling, and it reduced the amount of time your furnace is on. Both cut down the ventilation that is needed to remove the moisture produced by cooking, bathing, washing, etc. As a result, the humidity builds up to the point where condensation forms on cool surfaces like windows and walls. Condensation, in turn, promotes the growth of mildew.

The humidity must have been close to the condensation point before the ceiling was insulated, and it is possible that there are sources of moisture you can eliminate – a damp basement, for instance, or too many houseplants. In most cases, however, the only remedy is to replace some of the lost ventilation. The simplest way to do this is by opening a couple of windows a bit. But to avoid cold drafts you can simply install an exhaust fan in the bathroom and/or kitchen, where most household humidity originates. If you have a warm air furnace you can install a 4 in. or 5 in. duct to bring outside air directly to the cold air return side of the furnace. This allows the air to be filtered and heated before it is distributed to the rooms.

Of course this will use a little more heat, but I can tell you this will cost a lot less than the damage the excess humidity can do to your house in peeling paint, rotting wood and ruined insulation, not to mention the mildew damage you are already experiencing.

INSULATION SHEATHING

My builder wants to use semi-rigid fibreglass sheathing on the outside of our frame walls instead of ½ in. plywood. Will this provide as much structural support for the walls?

This is certainly not as strong as ½ in. plywood, but it doesn't have to be. Sheathing is not required to supply structural support – the framework does that. The fibreglass panels increase the insulation value of the walls, however, and that is why they are now widely used.

DON'T SEAL STORM WINDOWS

We have the old type of storm windows with wooden frames that have three holes at the bottom. For better insulation I put foam-type weatherstripping around the edges of the storm windows before I installed them this year, and then applied caulking around the outside edge. I also filled the holes in the frame with fibreglass wool and sealed them with tape. Now we are getting a lot of condensation on the inside of the storm windows. What did I do wrong?

The holes are put there for a purpose. Some ventilation is required behind a storm window to remove the humid household air that inevitably leaks past the inside window. If this is not done, the moisture in the air will condense on the cold storm windows, and that is what is happening now. The correct place for the weatherstripping is around the *inside* window. This will prevent household air from reaching the storm window, and it will also reduce heat loss. But you cannot stop this air leakage entirely, so some ventilation is still needed in the space between the two windows. Remove a little weatherstripping from the top of the storm window and open at least one of the holes at the bottom.

TOO MUCH INSULATION

Is there such a thing as having too much insulation? We have R30 in our attic now and are wondering if it would pay us to bring it up to R40.

Adding insulation will always reduce heat loss. But there's a catch. The value of each added inch of insulation diminishes as the thickness increases. The first inch saves a lot of heat; the second inch saves only half as much; the third inch reduces the remaining heat loss by one-third, and so on. The amount of heat you are loosing is reduced all the time, of course, and adding more insulation only saves a fraction of that. Eventually you will reach the point where the saving is less than the interest you would earn by just leaving the money in the bank.

At present and predicted fuel costs, R30 is close to the economical maximum amount of insulation for walls and ceilings, in my opinion. (Unless you're building a new house, that is, when it costs much less to insulate.) The money would be better spent, I think, insulating the basement walls, or installing caulking and weatherstripping to reduce air leakage.

DOES SUPERINSULATION PAY?

We are planning a new house and are thinking of having it built to the high insulton, low energy standards of the R2000 program that the government is promoting. Can you tell me if the added cost of such construction will really pay for itself by the reduced cost of heating and other energy consumption?

The federal government and the Canadian Home Builders' Association have been monitoring the cost and performance of the R2000 homes very carefully. Figures released this year show that the cost of the extra insulation and other energy-saving features *in excess of present building code requirements* has averaged $6300 per house. The average energy saving, on the other hand, works out to about $360 a year. That sounds impressive, but it is only about half the cost of carrying an additional $6300 on the mortgage at 10% interest. The payments on this would be $680 a year, for a net *loss* of $320 a year. (Even if you have the cash, you must still count the interest the $6300 would earn if you left it in government bonds or other secure investment.)

I have always been a strong advocate of adequate insulation, which many older homes still lack, but the money saved by insulation decreases with each added inch, and ultimately reaches the point where the cost of more insulation is greater than the energy saving it will achieve. I can find no figures that justify the cost of building superinsulated, low energy homes like the R2000. Residential building standards have been upgraded considerably in recent years, and are now about as good as they need to be for personal comfort and the economical use of insulation and energy.

INSULATING ROUGH STONE WALLS

Our old house has rough stone foundation walls. The basement is quite dry and we would like to add some living space down there, but can't figure out how to insulate the very uneven stone walls. Foamboard insulation won't fit at all, and an insulated frame wall would have many gaps behind it.

The best way to insulate a wall like this is with polyurethane foam. This is a highly rated insulating material – 2 in. (50mm) of it equals 3½ in. (90mm) of fibreglass – but it must be applied with industrial spray equipment. Firms that do this work can be found in the Yellow Pages under Insulation Materials.

Polyurethane foam is flammable and should be covered with a protective coating or fire barrier of some kind. A spray-on, cement-based stucco is one treatment. But if you want a smooth wall surface suitable for painting or papering, you can build a 2x4 frame wall in front of the insulated stone wall and panel this with gypsumboard.

INSULATION VALUE OF AIR SPACE

When adding a second pane of glass for extra insulation, as in a storm window, what is the most effective spacing? To put the question another way, does the insulation value of the air space continue to increase as it gets larger?

The insulation value of the air space between two panes of glass increases only slightly from ⅛ in. up to ¾ in. (3mm - 19mm), when it reaches its maximum level of a little less than R1, equal to about a third of an inch (8mm) of fibreglass batting. When the air space is larger than ¾ in., convection currents in the cavity counteract the insulation value by carrying heat from the warm inside pane to the cold outside pane – by cooling the inside pane, in other words. The only way to increase the insulation value with a larger air space is to divide it into two smaller spaces with a third pane.

INSULATION VALUE OF GLASS BLOCKS

I have obtained some reclaimed glass construction blocks that I hope to use in future renovations to my home. How does the insulation value of this material compare to conventional double- or triple-glazed windows?

Glass blocks are back in style again. They don't have much insulation value, however. A 4 in. thick clear block is rated at just R1.8, the same as a single pane plus a storm window, or a sealed, double-glazed thermal window with a ½ in. air space. A triple-glazed window is rated at R2.8, a lot better than the 4 in. block. The large air space really doesn't help, because it allows air currents to circulate inside the block and carry heat from one glass face to the other. Such air currents can't develop in a narrow air space.

INSULATION VALUE OF LOGS

We are thinking of having a log house built by a firm that specializes in this type of construction. The walls would be made of softwood logs about 8 in. (200mm) in diameter, with a notched joint between them packed with fibreglass wool to prevent air leakage. They tell me that this will provide much more insulation than standard house construction. Is this correct?

I'm afraid not. Wood is a beautiful material and I would love to own a log house, but wood is not a very good insulation material. The log construction you described would have less than one-half the insulation value of a standard wood frame wall insulated to present building code requirements.

Proponents of log construction often claim that wood has special qualities that make it a superior insulation material, but the scientific evidence does not support them. As insulation, wood behaves no differently than other materials used for this purpose. It slows down the rate of heat transfer from a warm area to a cold area because of all the tiny air cells it contains.

Internationally accepted standards for the measurement of this resistance to heat flow (or R value) have been in existence for many years, and are used by scientists everywhere to determine the insulation value of all materials, including wood. The accepted insulation value for the common construction softwoods is R1.25 per inch.

The average thickness of a wall made of 8 in. logs is about 6 in. Allowing for the insulation value of the inside and outside air films, this means that your log walls will have an average insulation value of about R8.5. The building code requires a minimun of R15 in wood frame walls – R3 to R4 in the construction material plus R12 in added insulation.

Builders of log houses argue that the insulation value of wood increases as the outside temperature drops. Indeed it does, very slightly, but so does every other insulation material. They also refer to a study done a few years ago by the Eastern Forest Products Labratory of the Canadian Forest Service that seemed to support such an idea. Subsequent investigation showed that the test methods were faulty, however. The study was discontinued and the report was never published. So even Canada's leading wood scientists agree that wood is not a very good insulation material.

But I would still build that log house, if I were you, even though it may cost a little more to heat than you expected. The other attractions of a log home will outweigh this small disadvantage.

INSULATION VALUE OF PATIO DOORS

We have a frame house and would like to install sliding patio doors in the north wall of our kitchen, opening to a wood deck. Which type of patio door would save the most heat; wood or aluminum?

You would lose a fair amount of heat through an uninsulated aluminum door frame, but the best aluminum doors (and windows) are now made with a layer of insulation, called a "thermal break", between the outside and inside sections of the metal frame. A solid wood frame has a little more insulation value than this, but not enough to make any significant difference in your heating bills.

Most of the heat is lost through the glass area, and the best insulation will be achieved with a unit that has two pairs of sliding doors, both with sealed, double-glazed thermal windows with a half-inch air space. But even this has much less insulation than an insulated frame wall, so whatever you do you are going to loose some heat. This is a small price to pay, however, for the convenience and pleasure you will get from opening the kitchen to the deck and garden. And in very cold weather you can reduce the heat loss by attaching panels of 1 in. foamboard to the inside of the doors. Covered with a decorative fabric, these can even be made quite attractive.

INSULATION VALUE OF SIDING

We need to have new siding put on our house and would like to know which kind provides the most insulation value: wood, metal or vinyl.

None of these provides enough insulation to have any significant effect on your heat loss, but wood is a little better than either unbacked metal or vinyl siding. Aluminum siding is often sold with a foam plastic or fibreboard backing, but this is put there mainly to reinforce the soft metal. The insulation value of the thin backing is minimal – no more than R2. The best way to insulate your walls is to have at least one inch of foamboard applied to the walls before the siding is put on.

WILL IT PAY TO INSULATE THE WALLS?

Our one-storey home is frame construction with stucco on three walls and cedar siding on the fourth. There is 2 in. of fibreglass insulation in the walls and about 4 in. in the ceiling. I have noticed houses being sheathed with blue foamboard insulation and then covered with vinyl siding. Would it pay me to have this done?

Your walls presently have an insulation value of R10 or R11. Adding 1 in. of this foamboard (the amount they usually put under siding) will bring the insulation value to about R15 and decrease the heat loss through the walls by about one-third.

You are probably losing about 25% of your heat through the walls now, so you can figure you will save about 8% on your annual heating costs by adding the foamboard and siding. If this will pay back the cost of the work in 10 years or less, at today's fuel prices, the job is worth doing. But I don't think it will.

As far as fuel savings are concerned, you would be better off if you added R20 insulation to your ceiling and then insulated the walls in your basement, which probably account for as much heat loss as the walls upstairs, but are a lot easier and cheaper to insulate.

MUST INSULATION ALWAYS "PAY"?

You have stated in your column several times that it does not always pay to add insulation to your house, that it may cost more than it saves. Seems to me you are overlooking the value of conserving our national energy resources. Doesn't this justify the cost of adding more insulation to our homes?

When I tell a reader that adding insulation in a particular situation will take a long time just to pay for itself in fuel savings, I am simply giving him (or her) the facts. Your concern about national energy conservation overlooks the fact that it takes a lot of energy to produce insulation. Fibreglass, for instance, is made in huge blast furnaces that consume a great deal of energy. Surely it is wasteful to use such insulation in places where it may save less fuel than it took to produce it. Only when the added insulation will reduce fuel consumption enough to pay for itself within a reasonable time (less than 10 years, certainly) can it be considered a benefit to either the homeowner or the country.

VAPOR BARRIER UNDER ATTIC INSULATION

Two summers ago I had loose insulation blown into my attic. I have since been told that a vapor barrier should have been laid down first to stop moisture collecting in the insulation. It is said that this will eventually rot the ceiling joists. Do I have to move all the insulation and put a vapor barrier down?

Theoretically, yes, but it is rarely done. And you should not have any problems unless your house is excessively humid during the winter – dripping windows, wet walls, etc. (for remedies see Condensation).

You should make sure you have plenty of ventilation in the attic, however – at least one square foot of open vent for every 300 square feet of ceiling. Vent openings should be located along the eaves and near the peak of the roof in order to get good air circulation.

VAPOR BARRIER UNDER COTTAGE FLOOR

I built an addition to my holiday home and insulated the floor by putting 6 in. batts up between the joists, then applying a plastic vapor barrier and holding it all in place with ¼ in. plywood. Under this is a crawlspace about 18 in. deep. Now I've been told that this is not the right way to do it. If that is so, how can I correct it?

The only thing wrong, as far as I can see, is that the vapor barrier should be on top of the insulation, not under it. This could trap condensation within the insulation.

Unfortunately, there is no easy way to correct this. The best remedy is to remove the plywood, vapor barrier and insulation and replace them in the proper order. Cut strips of vapor barrier 12 in. wider than the space between the joists, push them up under the floor and staple them to the sides of the joists. Then insert the batts and hold them in place with 15 in. lengths of coathanger wire wedged between the joists. Replace the plywood to keep stray animals

from using the batts as nesting material. Or better still, use ¼ in. wire screen to provide ventilation under the insulation while still protecting it from small animals.

But if you can keep the indoor humidity low enough in winter to prevent condensation on the windows (by keeping the cottage ventilated) you may not need to go to this much trouble. It may be enough just to ventilate the floor cavity by drilling ½ in. holes through the plywood and vapor barrier about every 8 in. between the joists. Or you can cut fewer and larger holes and cover them with wire screen.

IS SHEATHING A VAPOR BARRIER?

I am planning to build a house with 2x6 frame walls filled with fibreglass batts and covered with a vapor barrier and drywall panelling on the inside. This will provide R20 in insulation value. I would like to add another R10 with 2 in. of Styrofoam SM sheathing on the outside, but my carpenter tells me this will act as a second vapor barrier and trap moisture inside the wall. Is this correct?

No. By itself, Styrofoam *is* classed as Type 2 vapor barrier, but when it is applied as sheathing in 2 ft x 8 ft sheets, the joints provide all the ventilation that is required. This type of sheathing is now widely used and is approved by all building codes.

NOISE

BED SQUEAKING

What can I do to stop my daughter's bed from squeaking every time she moves? The noise seems to come from the spot where the side rail joins the headboard, but I can't see what's causing it.

If the connecting parts are metal, apply two or three drops of machine oil. If they are wood, use one of the white powder lubricants that come in a small plastic spray tube, available at any hardware store. Usually this will do it, but if the source of the squeak can't be reached this way, you will have to remove the mattress and box spring and unfasten the side rails. Wooden rails usually hook into a hidden slot in the leg of the headboard; to remove, place a scrap of wood underneath the side rail and hit it upwards with a hammer.

CANE CHAIR SEAT SQUEAKS

I have a high-backed chair with a cane seat and back. It was re-caned about a year ago and now squeaks very badly. Is there any way to stop this?

Soak the cane thoroughly with a wet sponge or cloth, then let it dry. This will tighten the cane webbing and should stop the squeaks.

THE DRIPPING GHOST

Whenever we turn on the hot water tap in the bathroom sink we hear a dripping sound in the wall behind it. We have never seen any sign of water in the wall, however, or any leak in the basement ceiling underneath it. Should we have the wall opened to see where the drip is going?

I don't think the dripping sound is due to water leakage. It is caused by the expansion of the pipe inside the wall when the hot water runs through it, causing it to rub against the woodwork or a supporting bracket in a jerking motion that sounds exactly like water dripping inside the wall.

The only cure is to open the wall and bend the pipe away from the wall, or wedge something behind it, but this is a drastic remedy for what is really just a momentary annoyance that is not causing any trouble. Knowing this, perhaps, will be enough to put your mind at rest.

NOISY DRAINS

Whenever any of the drains in the bathroom on the second floor are used, it sounds like Niagara Falls in the room below. The 3 in. plastic drain pipe comes down inside a wall, then runs under the floor about 10 ft and joins the main cast iron drain stack. Would it help to remove the wall panelling and pack fibreglass wool around the plastic pipe?

That bend in the pipe where it turns under the floor is the cause of the problem, I think. A vertical drain pipe is relatively quiet, because water doesn't fall free down the center of it as you would expect; it spirals down the inside surface of the pipe, leaving the centre open for air to escape. The noise you hear is produced when the falling water meets the right-angle turn under the floor. I don't think there's any way to change this, but wrapping the pipe with fibreglass wool might help a bit.

DUCT NOISES

For the past two winters, ever since we bought our house, we have been bothered by nightly banging sounds in the warm air heating system. People tell us it's caused by the expansion and contraction of the pipes and we'll get used to it, but I don't understand how this works and we're not getting used to it. Can you explain the problem and give us a remedy?

If you've ever used an oil can you know how it makes a snapping sound when you press the bottom. That's how sheet metal ductwork produces noise as it expands and contracts with changes in temperature. As a mattter of fact, tinsmiths refer to this as "oil-canning".

It can be stopped simply be wedging something against the side of the duct – or even by giving it a sharp blow with a hammer – but first you have to find exactly where the noise is coming from. If this is more than 6 ft from the furnace you can wedge a piece of wood or anything else against the duct to keep it from snapping. If it's closer than that you'll have to use a fireproof material, or use a hammer to dent the metal slightly. Where the offending duct is inside a wall or floor, you may be able to reach inside it with a hammer. If not, you'll have to open the wall or ceiling to get at it.

EXHAUST DUCT RATTLES

The bathroom fan outlet on the side of our house rattles very loudly when the wind blows. It is right beside our bedroom and keeps us awake at night. How can we stop this?

It will be the hinged flap that is rattling. All you need to do is add a little weight to the flap – just enough to hold it down against the wind, but not enough to keep it from opening when the fan is operating. The easiest way to do this is glue a metal washer to the bottom of the flap, using caulking compound or silicone adhesive. A few tests will show you what size of washer you need.

NOISE IN ELECTRIC FURNACE

When the heating elements in my electric furnace come on they make a rattling noise. It seems to come from the ceramic rings that support the heating coils. Is there anything I can do to stop this?

The noise could be caused by loose rings, but it is not advisable to try to tighten these yourself; they break very easily. It could also be caused by the blower fan running too fast. You need an expert to check that, too. Most likely, however, the vibration is produced by a defective heating element. Ask the furnace supplier to send a serviceman to check it.

A SHRIEKING FAUCET

When we turn on the hot water faucet in our vanity sink we get a high-pitched shrieking noise. It is the only faucet in the house that does this. What is the cause and how can we stop it?

Technically, this is known as "cavitation noise", and it's caused by water being forced through a restricted opening, causing the velocity to increase and the pressure to drop. This releases gas bubbles that produce the screeching sound as they collapse. The action is even strong enough to corrode metal.

The restriction may be no more than a burr around the inside of a copper pipe where it was cut. Tube cutters include a reamer that is supposed to be used to remove this, but amateur plumbers, and some professionals, sometimes forget to do this. The pipe connections will have to be taken apart to find and remove the restriction in the faucet line.

SQUEAKS IN CARPETED FLOOR

The upstairs floor in our house squeaks very badly. I understand that I can stop this by driving nails through the subflooring into the joists, but the floor is covered with wall-to-wall carpeting and I don't know where the joists are. What can I do?

Normally you can locate the joists simply by tapping on the floor and listening for the solid sound, but you can't do that through a carpet. Instead, you'll have to drill a small hole in the floor and use a wire probe to find the joists.

Spread the pile apart with your fingers and drill a 3/16 in. hole through the carpet backing, underlay and subfloor (probably 1/2 in. plywood). Bend a 17 in. length of coathanger wire into a Z shape with a bottom leg 9 in. long, a 3 in. upright section and a 5 in. handle section on the top. Push the long section through the hole in the floor and rotate it with the handle section. When it strikes a joist, lay a pencil on the carpet to indicate the exact direction the wire is pointing.

Remove the wire and position it on top of the carpet at the angle indicated by the pencil. The end of the wire will show where it met the joist. A nail driven 3/4 in. over from this should hit the centre of the joist. Other joists will run parallel to this every 16 in.. Use 2 in. spiral finishing nails at the places where the floor is squeaking. Drive the heads through the carpet with a nail-set. The pile will close over the hole.

NOISY FLOORS vs HUMIDITY

Every winter we have a problem with squeaking floors. A few years ago we had the wall-to-wall carpet taken up and more nails put in the plywood subfloor, but the problem continued. Then we put in a humidifier, thinking that our electric furnace was causing the air to be too dry. The humidity is now high enough for the windows to drip, but the floors still squeak. What else can we do?

The squeaking is caused by movement of the subfloor when it is walked on, and can usually be remedied by nailing the plywood to the joists with ringed flooring nails. Dry air is generally the cause, certainly, but in your case I think the problem is *too much* humidity, making the plywood swell and buckle slightly.

Electric heat is no drier than oil or gas heat. In fact it has the opposite effect, because it does not provide the ventilation produced by a fuel-burning furnace, and therefore allows the humidity created by cooking, washing, bathing, etc., to build up. If you turn the humidifier off and ventilate the house a little more – enough to stop condensation forming on the windows – I think you will see an improvement in the noise problem.

FLUORESCENT FIXTURES vs RADIO

I recently replaced three incandescent lighting fixtures in my basement with new fluorescent fixtures. After the lights have been on for about 15 minutes we get a very loud and annoying interference on our radios. If the fluorescent lights are switched off, the noise stops immediately.

Sometimes this can be stopped simply by reversing the leads to the fluorescent fixtures – switching the black and white wires, in other words. You should also check the wiring to make sure that the fixture housing is properly grounded (if it isn't, it can also cause starting problems).

If these steps don't help, then the ballasts must be defective. Either buy new ballasts (make sure you get the exact same type) or take the fixtures back to the supplier for a replacement. Most manufacturers give a 3-year warranty on fluorescent ballasts.

HEAT PUMP NOISE

I had an all-electric heat pump installed in my house last fall. To prevent noise problems, I had the compressor unit located 40 ft from the house, but we are getting a pulsating, throbbing sound from the furnace unit in the basement, and the noise is transmitted through the house by the ductwork. The serviceman says this is a common problem when there is a long run between the house and the compressor, and suggests that it cannot be corrected.

It is a recognized problem, all right, but there are remedies for it. The sound of the compressor is transmitted by the refrigerant in the pipes that come into the basement, and these may not have been installed correctly. They should be supported by special flexible, cushioned, metal hangers that keep the vibrations from being transmitted to the framework of the house. If rigid fasteners were used in your installation, they should be replaced.

The vibrations can also be kept outside the house by installing a special fitting simply called a "muffler", in the refrigerant line between the discharge side of the compressor and the 3-way valve. This device is now standard equipment on most heat pump compressors, but if yours does not have one the serviceman can easily install it.

HOUSE FRAME CREAKS

Our 12-year-old, 3-bedroom, frame house makes strange noises. Cracking sounds are heard periodically throughout the house. They start in one corner and travel across the house, sometimes loud, sometimes soft, but always annoying. Strangely enough, however, no cracks have appeared. Can you tell us what causes this noise and what we can do about it?

I can tell you the cause, but I don't know of any cure. The sounds are probably caused by movement within the framework of the house, probably due to changes in temperature, humidity or wind pressure. You can get a clue to the cause by noting when it happens. If it occurs in the evening, for instance, a drop in outdoor temperature is the most likely cause of the sound. Humidity alters slowly, but it could be the cause if the noises only start when the weather changes dramatically. The most likely cause, however, is wind pressure, which should be easy to check.

The only remedy would be to brace or reinforce the house envelope, and I don't know of any practical way to do that unless you want to put new sheathing and siding on the house.

OIL FURNACE BACKFIRES

We had a new oil furnace installed over a year ago, and it has always had an annoying noise problem. Every time it comes on there is a small explosion, like a car backfiring, sometimes loud enough to wake us up at night. The heating company that put it in says the furnace is OK and there's nothing they can do about the noise.

This is usually due to delayed ignition, which can be caused by a number of things. The spark electrodes may be dirty or incorrectly placed. Or there may be insufficient burner draft. Sometimes the backfiring can be corrected simply by putting a smaller nozzle on the burner. Most furnaces are oversized, anyway, and reducing the size of the nozzle will also improve heat efficiency.

WHINING NOISE IN RADIATORS

Last summer, on the advice of our plumber, we had a pump added to our old gravity hot water heating system to circulate the water more efficiently. The house temperature does stay much steadier now, but we are disturbed by a high-pitched whining noise that comes from all the radiators. The plumber says this is just the sound of the pump and it's perfectly natural. We think it's unnatural. Do you have any suggestions?

This is probably something called "velocity noise", caused when an oversized pump is put on an old hot water heating system that has a large water capacity. The plumber miscalculated the size of the pump, in other words.

The best remedy is to replace the pump with a smaller one but that would be expensive unless the plumber will make the exchange. If there is a valve on the discharge side of the pump (the boiler side, usually), you can simply close this slightly to reduce the flow of water below the noise level. If there isn't such a valve, it would be cheaper to install one than put in a new pump. A small and relatively inexpensive "balancing valve" is all you need. Another simple remedy, recommended by a leading pump manufacturer, is to have the impeller in the pump cut down to a smaller size.

NOISY REFRIGERATOR

My 10-year-old refrigerator has begun making a banging noise when the motor goes off. Other than that it works fine. I am handy with tools and would like to know if there is anything I can do to correct this problem myself so it won't keep waking me up in the night.

A loose mounting bolt may be causing the compressor to shake when it slows down. Unplug the refrigerator and move it out from the wall so you can remove the service panel at the back. The compressor is usually mounted on rubber pads and held down with four bolts. You may only have to tighten the bolts, but sometimes the rubber mounts have deteriorated and must be replaced. Get replacement mounting pads from the local service company or distributor who handles this make of refrigerator. Unscrew one mounting bolt at a time and raise the compressor just enough to slip out the old mounting pad and replace it with a new one. Put the bolt back and go on to the next one.

WINTER ROOF NOISE

My townhouse has a flat roof. During the winter, whenever the temperature drops below freezing we hear loud noises from the roof. They sound like hammer blows. What causes this and what can we do about it?

This is probably due to water ponding on the roof and then freezing. The stresses this builds up in the roof and ice can cause sharp cracking noises like those you describe. They are frequently heard by top floor residents in apartment buildings, too.

Check the roof after a rain to see where and how much the water is ponding, take some photographs of it, then ask at least three roofing contractors to quote a price for correcting the drainage.

NOISY SPACE HEATER

We installed a gas-fired space heater in our country home and it does its job very well. The only problem we have with it is the loud bang it makes when it begins to heat up, and again when it cools off. My husband says: "If it's working, don't fix it," but I find the noise very disturbing.

This is a common problem with many kinds of heating equipment. It is called "oil-canning," and is caused when a sheet of metal is heated, expands, and snaps in or out like the bottom of an oil can when you press on it. It snaps back again when the metal cools and contracts, of course.

There are several things you can do to stop the noise. The heater may be supported unevenly by the floor; if so, just propping up one of the corners may correct the problem. Otherwise, try to find which sheet of metal is popping when it is heated. If this happens to be held in place with screws, try tightening or loosening them. If this does not work, hit the metal with a hammer, just hard enough to dent it slightly, Not a very sophisticated remedy, perhaps, but it works.

SQUEAKY STAIRS

Some of the stair treads leading to our second floor bedrooms squeak very badly. The trouble is that I can't get at them because they are fully carpeted on top, and the underside, over the basement stairway, is completely covered. What can I do to stop them squeaking?

Usually, all you need to do is nail the front of the noisy tread to the riser that supports it, and this isn't difficult. Simply spread the carpet pile apart and drive a 2¼ in. spiral finishing nail between the tufts, then use a nailset to drive the head down through the carpet and into the riser. If necessary, the same thing can be done at the side of the tread, but the nail will have to be driven in at a 45° angle there.

NOISY GAS WATER HEATER

Our 33-gallon gas-fired hot water tank thumps and bangs as if it's going to explode when the washing machine is being used. Can you tell me what's causing this?

It's probably due to a buildup of scale on the bottom of the tank. The washing machine draws a lot of water from the tank, causing the burner to stay on for a long time. This causes the water temperature under the scale to build up close to the boiling point, causing vapor bubbles to form. These collapse with an exploding sound when they reach the cooler water above the scale. It's the same process that causes the popping sound you hear in a kettle as it nears the boiling point.

Lowering the temperature of the water should stop the trouble. Somewhere between 140° and 150°F is high enough. It would also be a good idea to drain a pail of water from the valve at the bottom of the tank in order to remove some of the scale. If the tank has scaled badly, however, it probably should be replaced.

ELECTRIC WATER HEATER HISSES

The electric water heater at my summer place makes a hissing, sizzling sound when the power comes on. It is a standard 40-gallon tank with two elements. What would cause this?

It could be a loose electrical connection. Turn off the power to the circuit that controls the water heater and leave it off until the problem has been found and corrected. To check it yourself, remove the panels that give access to the heating elements, then loosen one terminal screw and remove the wire. If it is blackened or corroded, cut off the bare wire, strip the insulation off the next half inch, re-insert in the terminal block and tighten the screw. Check and replace one wire at a time like this so you don't get them mixed up. When all the wires have been checked and tightened, restore power to the water heater to make sure the noise has stopped. If not, you might need a new thermostatic control. Disconnect the power again and call in an electrician. Or do this in the beginning if you don't want to work on the wiring.

BANGING IN WATER PIPES

Sometimes when we turn off a tap quickly a loud banging noise can be heard in the pipes. I am afraid one of them is going to burst. What can we do to stop this noise?

A solid column of water carries sound like a metal bar. When the water is shut off suddenly in certain types of faucets and washing machine valves, it's like hitting the end of the bar with a hammer. The phenomenon is known as "water hammer", in fact. The remedy is to put a sealed air chamber in the water pipe close to the offending tap to cushion the shock wave. A vertical length of pipe capped at the top will do, but diaphram-type "shock arrestors" are available at most plumbing supply stores. Both types require a tee fitting in the supply pipe close to the tap.

RATTLING SOUND IN WATER PIPES

We live in a charming old 3-storey house with just one problem. Every time we turn on a tap – hot or cold, on any floor – there is a steady rattling sound in the pipes.

This could be caused by loose washers in the taps, but it's unlikely that you would have a loose washer in every tap. The other possibility is that your water pressure is too high, causing the pipes to vibrate. If you have a pressure-reducing valve in the supply line where it enters the house, this can be adjusted very easily. If you don't have such a valve, a plumber can install one. But first check to see if you can locate the vibrating pipe. Trace the pipes that lead to the upper floors and hold onto them as someone opens a tap. If you can find the pipe that's vibrating you may be able to secure it or wedge something beside it to keep it from moving.

ODORS

BARN ODOR IN HOUSE?

It was our intention to convert a small log barn into a vacation cabin suitable for year-round use, but someone has told us that a building that has housed animals will never be suitable for human occupation. This barn hasn't been used for over 25 years, but we are told that animal odors will come out of the wood as soon as it's heated. Is this true?

That suggestion will come as a surprise to the many people who have converted old barns into charming homes, or who have used authentic barnboard to panel the walls of their city homes. I have visited, photographed and written about a lot of beautiful homes that once were barns, and no one ever complained about such a problem. Such odors are biodegradable, in any case, and I'm sure they will have disappeared many years ago.

ODOR FROM BASEMENT FLOOR DRAIN

My house is about 30 years old and I am having trouble with a sewer odor coming from the basement floor drain. I tried bleach and lye (at different times) but they didn't do any good.

Like all the drains in your house, the basement floor drain has a U-shaped trap below the opening. If the drain is used regularly, the trap will always have some water in it, and this will prevent sewer gases from getting into the house. A floor drain is seldom used these days, however, and the water in the trap evaporates.

63

The simple remedy is to pour a couple of quarts of water down the drain every month or so to keep the odor trap closed. If this doesn't work it will mean that there is a leak in the trap connection. To repair that, a plumber will have to open the floor around the drain and replace or re-connect the trap. He should also install a special tap in the laundry tub; this will run a little water into the drain trap whenever the tap is used. These are now required in all new homes.

REMOVING FUEL OIL SMELL

While I was away from my house for a month the fuel pump in my oil furnace sprang a leak and oil soaked into the concrete floor. I used sawdust to soak up the spill and got the pump fixed, but the smell of the fuel oil is still very strong. What can I do to get rid of it?

First clean the floor with one of the grease removers sold at hardware and auto supply stores – Gunk, Dunk and Polyclens are three common brands. Spray or pour one of these on the oil stain, brush in well, let stand for 15 minutes or so, then apply water, brush again and hose off. Repeat if necessary.

There are also a number of deodorizers on the market that are made specially for use with fuel oil, and you should be able to get one from your oil supplier, or any heating equipment supply company. Brands include Banz-Odor, Odorout and Neutroda. These all come in spray cans and are easy to use. They should keep the odor under control until the house can be aired out properly during the summer.

OIL SMELL FROM FURNACE

There is a smell of fuel oil around our furnace, but I can't see any sign of an oil leak. It is most noticeable just after the furnace comes on. What would cause this?

It is probably cause by a "blowback" that expels a small puff of oil smoke into the furnace room. This is due to delayed ignition, perhaps because the spark electrodes are dirty or improperly placed, or because there is not the right draft pressure through the burner. Sometimes it can be corrected just by opening the viewing port over the burner slightly, or installing a smaller nozzle. (Most furnaces are oversized, anyway, and a smaller nozzle will improve burner efficiency.) Your furnace serviceman should have no trouble correcting this problem.

KITCHEN ODORS

I do a lot of cooking and am partial to spices, so have a problem with kitchen odors spreading through the rest of the house. We installed a ductless vent hood over the stove but it hasn't helped very much, if at all. Should I install an exhaust fan in an outside wall or put it in the ceiling and run the ductwork up through the roof? The kitchen is 10 ft x 12 ft. What size fan do we need?

Ductless range hoods provide no ventilation at all, of course. They merely pass the cooking fumes through a grease filter that removes some of the oils, and a charcoal filter that absorbs a certain amount of the odors. They are not nearly as effective as an exhaust fan.

The best place for this is in the range hood itself, provided there is room for it and also space for the ductwork. The next best place for the exhaust fan would be in an outside wall close to the stove, with no ductwork to impede the air flow. A ceiling fan would be the next choice, with ductwork running between the ceiling joists to an outside wall if it's a 2-storey house, or across the attic to a vent in the roof overhang if it's a 1-storey house. Running the ductwork straight up through the roof isn't a very good way to do it, since condensation inside the vertical duct may drip back through the ceiling fan. If this is the only practical location for the vent, however, wrap the duct with insulation batts where it goes through the cold attic.

Exhaust fans are rated according to the number of cubic feet of air they move per minute (CFM). A range hood fan should have a rating of at least 40 CFM per foot of hood – a 36 in. hood requires a 120 CFM fan, in other words. A wall or ceiling fan should have a CFM rating equal to twice the area of the kitchen in square feet – or 240 CFM in your case.

OZONE SMELL FROM ELECTROSTATIC FILTER

Last winter we had an electrostatic air filter installed in our gas furnace, and shortly after that we began to notice a very unpleasant odor. A friend who happened to drop in at that time asked, as soon as he came in, if we had installed an electrostatic air filter. He said he recognized the odor of ozone produced by the filter and told us this wasn't healthy. The company that installed the unit says the ozone smell is natural and perfectly safe, but we're still concerned. Can you tell us whether we should be?

Ozone is an active form of oxygen that is produced in nature by electrical storms and ultraviolet light. It is also produced by any electric spark or similar discharge, and is the source of the "electricity smell" commonly noticed where electric motors or generators are running.

Too much ozone can irritate eyes and respiratory passages, and health authorities recommend an indoor level of no more than .050 parts per million, which is slightly higher than the average level of ozone in city air, according to U.S. studies. The concentration of ozone in a home with an electrostatic air cleaner ranges from one-tenth to one-fifth of the recommended maximum, but some people are more sensitive to ozone than others and may notice it at even lower concentrations.

There is no practical way to measure the ozone level in your house, but there are several ways it can be lowered. One is to have an activated charcoal filter put in the air cleaner. The company that installed it can do this. The filter will have to be replaced every few months. Another remedy is to have the wiring on the transformer in the air cleaner changed to reduce the voltage on the electrostatic filter element. This will also reduce the effectiveness of the unit slightly, however. The only other remedy is to stop using the air cleaner.

PET ODOR IN BASEMENT FLOOR

I rented my house to someone who, unknown to me, kept a large dog in the basement. There is a strong urine odor in several areas of the concrete floor. Detergents, bleach and airing have done some good, but the smell is still very bad. What can I do to get rid of it?

Pet stores sell a number of products for removing such odors, but one of the most effective treatments is a 15% solution of acetic acid. Any druggist will make this up for you if you tell him what it's for. He may suggest using vinegar, but this is only 5% acetic acid, which is not strong enough for the job. Depending on how much you are going to need, it might pay you to buy lab grade glacial acetic acid from a chemical supply house. You can get 500ml for less than $10, and this is enough to make 3.5 litres (3 quarts) of 15% solution. Glacial acetic acid is corrosive and must be handled with care, but the 15% solution is not hazardous.

SEPTIC TANK ODOR

About a year ago I moved into a house I built in a pleasant rural area. It has an approved septic tank disposal system. Both

last summer and this we have been troubled by a sewer-like smell on our patio whenever there is a slight breeze. A plumber has suggested putting an extension on the roof vent stack. Would this be the answer?

The odor will be coming from the plumbing vent pipe, all right, but I do not think you can extend this enough to make any difference. The problem is often caused by the use of a tee connection where the house drain enters the septic tank. If the top arm of the tee extends above the fluid level in the tank, sewer gases can escape back through the house drain to the vent stack on the roof, where air currents can bring it back to ground level. To prevent this, CSA septic tank standard CAN3-B66 recommends the use of an elbow fitting that is not open above the liquid level. If inspection shows that you have an open tee fitting there, the simple remedy is to place a heavy ceramic tile or similar object on top of the open tee.

It is possible, of course, that the odor is coming from a neighbor's vent stock. If so, tell *him* what the remedy is.

SEWER ODOR

We did some remodelling to our house that involved moving the laundry tubs in the basement to a new location. Now we get a sewer smell from the tub drains after they are emptied. Can you offer any suggestions as to what would cause this and what we can do about it?

The problem is in the U-shaped drain trap under the laundry tubs. There is supposed to be enough water in this at all times to prevent sewer gases from entering the house. To keep the water from being syphoned out of the trap every time the tub is emptied, it must be connected to an open vent pipe that goes up through the roof. Either this vent pipe has been disconnected from the laundry tub drain, or it is now too far away from it to serve its purpose.

A vent pipe must be located no more than 5 ft from a drain trap. If there is some reason why a vent pipe can't be connected within that distance of the laundry tubs now, you can use an automatic plumbing vent, a plastic one-way valve that attaches to the drain pipe just behind the trap. These are not approved for new construction, but you can install one in your own house. They're available at most plumbing supply stores for less than $10.

SEWER SMELL FROM FLOODED BASEMENT

During a recent storm our local drainage

system was flooded and water backed up into our basement. Fortunately there wasn't too much damage, but there is still an unpleasant sewer odor coming from the concrete floor. I've washed it with everything I can think of, including chlorine bleach.

Try a strong solution of lye. I suggest using one 9½ ounce (269 grams) can to a gallon of water. Apply this with a mop and leave it on the floor for about one hour before rinsing it off down the floor drain. Wear old shoes and clothes and be careful not to get the caustic solution on your skin. If you do, wipe it off immediately with a wet rag.

BAD ODOR IN HOT SHOWER

We have bought a house with a strange problem. The bathroom off the master bedroom has a shower stall the produces a sickening odor whenever hot water is used. There is no smell at all with a cold shower. I have checked the plumbing vent stack and the shower drain and can find nothing wrong with them.

The odor may come from hydrogen sulphide, the rotten egg gas, produced from sulphates in the water supply. The gas can be created by the action of a certain type of bacteria that thrive in the hot, oxygen-free environment of a water heater. The odor should be noticeable wherever you turn on a hot water tap, but it would certainly be a lot stronger if you were standing in a hot shower. And you wouldn't get it at all in a cold shower, of course.

One remedy for this problem is to remove the magnesium anode from the hot water tank completely (which will shorten the life of the tank). Another remedy is to replace it with an aluminum anode that will still provide protection against corrosion but doesn't offer such favorable conditions for the bacteria that produce the rotten egg odor. A third remedy is to install a sulphate filter on your water supply.

SMOKE SMELL FROM FIREPLACE

We have a problem with our fireplace. Even though I clean it out the day after having a fire in it, we keep getting the smell of smoke, ashes and burned wood in the house. Presumably this is from air coming down the chimney, although that has been cleaned, too. Would a rain cap on the chimney help?

A chimney-top damper would do more good than a rain cap. As the name indicates, this sits on top of the chimney and is controlled by a lever at the fireplace. Unlike the usual fireplace damper, it provides an almost airtight seal. Various models are available at stores that sell wood stoves and fireplaces.

The fact that air is being drawn *down* the unused chimney suggests that your house may be too tightly sealed, and there is a danger that the furnace is not getting all the air it needs. Opening a window in the furnace room might cure both problems.

BAD SMELL FROM HOT WATER

I have received conflicting advice about a problem concerning a rotten egg smell from our hot water. There doesn't seem to be any smell from the cold water. I have been told that the remedy is to remove the magnesium anode from the hot water tank, but others tell me that this will destroy the tank. I can't believe that it would do any good, anyway, because the tank had no anode at all for a couple of years and the smell was just as bad.

The cause of the odor is sulphur in the water. Heat promotes bacterial action that converts the sulphur to hydrogen sulphide, which smells like rotten eggs. Electrochemical action around the magnesium anode, which prevents the tanks from corroding, also stimulates the bacteria, and it has been found that some improvement can be achieved by replacing the magnesium anode with an aluminum one.

The best remedy, however, is to install a filter that will remove the sulphur from the water before it gets to the hot water tank. This is done by adding a little chlorine bleach to precipitate the sulphur, then passing the water through a filter bed that removes both the sulphur and the chlorine. The equipment is available from any company that sells water softeners.

PAINT PROBLEMS

ALLIGATORED PAINT

Last year I applied two coats of alkyd, semigloss paint to our kitchen walls, and now the finish has developed a random pattern of fine cracks that resembles alligator skin. What would cause this, and what can I do to corrrect it?

"Alligatoring" is the common trade term for this paint problem, which is often caused by painting over a glossy finish without roughening it first with sandpaper to provide a "tooth" for the new coat. In your case, however, it could be due to another common mistake – applying a second coat of oil-based or alkyd paint before the first one has dried completely, This keeps the first coat soft while the top coat is drying, which can cause the surface film to crack in this characteristic pattern.

If the alligatored paint is peeling, all coats must be removed entirely with a chemical paint stripper, which is a big job. But if it is firmly attached, you can overcome the problem by filling the cracks with a plaster patching material or drywall joint compound. This should be mixed to a sloppy consistency ("about the same as Pablum," one authority suggests) and applied with a broad putty knife or a square plastering trowel. When dry, smooth with fine sandpaper on a wood block, then apply another coat of filler to level the small depressions that are left when the first application dries (you will see these if you shine a light across the wall). Use the sanding block again to achieve a perfectly smooth wall surface, then apply an alkyd primer and repaint.

BLISTERING PAINT

We have always had trouble with paint blistering on our wood siding, but this year it got much worse. We would like to find out how to stop this before we paint again. The previous owner caulked all the siding boards, and we have scraped this out to let the walls breathe. What else should we do to stop the blistering?

The blistering is probably caused by moist household air getting into the wall cavity and condensing behind the siding during cool weather. This is very likely soaking the insulation in the walls, too, and eventually it will rot the wood framework as well.

You were right to remove the caulking on the siding to ventilate the walls, but what you need to do now is caulk *inside* the house. Remove the baseboards and caulk along the bottom of the outside walls. Take off the trim (the picture moulding) around the windows and inject urethane foam between the rough frame and the frame of the window itself. Seal around wiring and plumbing holes in the wall and in the basement ceiling directly underneath it. Insert foam pad air seals behind the cover plates on wall outlets and switches.

Something must have happened to increase the humidity in your house within the last couple of years. Perhaps the size of your family has increased, resulting in more baths, washing

and cooking. Or you may have added a humidifier, or disconnected a dryer vent. More likely, however, there has been some change that reduced the amount of ventilation the house gets during the winter. Weatherstripping and storm windows will do this. So will putting in a high efficiency furnace, because this does not draw as much air into the house as a conventional furnace does. Switching to electric heating reduces ventilation even more, because it completely eliminates the air infiltration provided by a fuel-burning furnace and chimney. One of these is surely the cause if you are also troubled with dripping windows during the winter months, because this is an unmistakable sign of excessive humidity. The best remedy is to put an exhaust fan in the bathroom or kitchen, the main sources of household moisture. (See also Condensation)

CEILING PEELING

A couple of years ago we bought a 35-year-old bungalow and painted all the rooms before we moved in. Some months later we noticed a crack in the paint on one of the ceilings. It gradually got bigger and pretty soon the paint came off in large pieces right down to the smooth, hard surface of the original plaster, which still seems to be in good condition. The same thing happened in other rooms. The salesman at the paint store says this was caused by dampness, but there is no sign of this on the ceiling or in the attic.

A number of people have written me about this problem and I have also experienced it myself. Paint experts I discussed it with have suggested a number of possible causes but no clearcut answers. Most paint failure is caused by moisture getting under the surface film so this is the standard explanation, but the facts don't always support this answer, as in your case.

In an older house this problem can be due to a buildup of too many paint layers. The last one can be the final straw that pulls the whole multilayered paint membrane off the smooth plaster. In such a case, of course, it is the first layer that fails, not the last one. The plaster may not have been perfectly dry when this was put on, which would have weakened the bond of this critical layer. Or the first coat could have been calcimine. This powdered casein paint was cheap and popular many years ago, and was still being used when your house was built, but it didn't provide a very good base for the latex paints that eventually replaced it.

Whatever the cause, the only remedy is to remove all the old paint down to the plaster. Most of it can be scraped off with a broad putty knife or similar tool. The rest can be softened with a hot-air gun or an electric paint remover, but these must be used with caution indoors.

If the old plaster is very smooth it should be roughened with #80 sandpaper and then dusted carefully before applying a flat latex paint.

REFINISHING PEELING CEILING

My roof leaked very badly about three years ago and the many layers of paint in the area of the ceiling that was wet have peeled off the plaster. Now I would like to repair it but I do not know how to fill the depression left by the flaking, multi-layered paint, which must be about 1/16-inch thick. Do I have to strip all the paint off the ceiling to get a smooth, paintable surface?

Use a putty knife to get under the edge of the loose paint layer and remove as much as you can. If the bare area is no more than two square feet or so in size you may be able to level it with one of the plaster patching materials and a rectangular 10 in. or 11 in. plaster trowel. With a little practice you should be able to spread the filler fairly smoothly. When dry, sand with #100 paper on a wood block and then apply a thin topping coat the same way. But if the area is fairly large you would be better off to get a plasterer to do it.

CRACKS IN NEW PAINT

My kitchen cupboard had been painted with an oil-based paint. Not knowing any better, I refinished it with a latex paint. The cupboard is now covered with a spiderweb of fine cracks. I've tried sanding and repainting, but the cracks still show. What should I do?

There's no reason why you can't apply latex over an oil-based paint. If the finish was glossy, however, it should have been sanded lightly first to provide a "tooth" for the new finish. I suspect this was the cause of your trouble.

To restore a smooth surface you must first fill the cracks. Use a 3 in. putty knife and any of the premixed crack fillers or spackling compounds. When the filler has dried, sand the surface lightly with fine paper on a block of wood, remove the sanding dust, then repaint with either latex or oil-based paint. Two coats may be necessary.

FLOOR PAINT BLISTERING

We recently purchased and moved into an 11-year-old house. Everything looked fine when we inspected it before buying, but a few days after we moved in we noticed that the paint on the basement floor was blistering. Under the blisters we found a dry white powder. Can you tell us what this is?

The blistering is caused by moisture seeping up through the concrete floor, due to insufficient drainage under it. The moisture brings with it dissolved mineral salts that are left inside the blisters when the water evaporates. Perhaps the former owners were aware of this problem and painted the floor to conceal it.

The only remedy is to improve the drainage. The cheapest way to do this is to put a sump pump in the floor, but the best remedy is to have a drainage contractor correct your present drainage system or install a new one.

IDENTIFYING PAINT

We recently purchased an older home and would like to repaint the exterior this summer. I have been told that we should use the same *kind* of paint that is on there now, latex or oil-based, but how can we determine which kind we have?

Most experts now agree that it does not make much difference as long as the present paint is firmly attached and has been properly cleaned. But a painter's trick for identifying paint is to apply a little nail polish remover to a test spot. Latex paint will be softened and rub off easily. An alkyd or oil-based paint will just be dulled slightly.

LINSEED OIL FINISH

Ten years ago my father and I built a cottage and covered it with cedar siding, which we finished with two coats of boiled linseed oil. The oil never dried properly and soon collected dirt and bugs. After a couple of years the surface began to turn black in places, as if mildewed. We tried scraping this off and applying more linseed oil, but within a year the black patches were back. How can we remove these and restore the natural wood finish?

You have discovered the disadvantages of linseed oil as a finish for exterior wood: it dries slowly and is hospitable to mildew and other molds. I know of no practical way to remove the finish and restore the natural wood. The best you can do is apply a flat paint in a color close to the wood tone you want. Scrub the siding first with a solution that will clean it and kill the mildew - 3 quarts of water, 1 quart of liquid laundry bleach and ½ cup of powdered dishwasher detergent. Then apply the paint of your choice (one of the so-called "solid stains" might be best).

MILDEW-RESISTANT PAINT

We live in a damp area that is close to trees, and are having a lot of trouble with mildew growing on our house paint. What is the best paint to use to prevent this?

All exterior house paints contain a fungicide that inhibits mildew growth, but most of these chemicals are also hazardous to humans. With the growing concern about exposure to such chemicals there has been an effort to cut down on their use, and I believe this is the main cause for the gradual increase in paint mildew problems that I have seen in my mail over the last few years.

Unfortunately, paint manufacturers do not give the consumer any information about the amount or kind of fungicide in their exterior house paints, so there is no way of knowing which brand is the most resistant to mildew. You can increase the mildew resistance of any paint, however, by adding a fungicide to it. One of the safest and easiest to use is Dettol antiseptic, which contains phenol, a very effective germicide and fungicide. This can be added to any latex, oil-based or alkyd paint at the rate of 15ml (1 tablespoon) per litre. Stir in thoroughly before using.

The present mildewed paint should be scrubbed clean first, however, with a solution of one part chlorine laundry bleach to three parts water, plus 60ml (¼ cup) of dishwasher detergent per litre of solution.

PAINT PEELING ON GARAGE

Our wood frame garage is used as a workshop and is heated in winter by a small wood stove. The painted siding peels very badly every year and must be scraped off and repainted. What can I do to prevent this?

The heat is causing moisture vapor inside the garage to migrate through the wood siding, where it condenses under the paint and causes it to peel. The remedy is to insulate the walls with 3½ in. fibreglass batts, cover them with polyethylene vapor barrier, then gypsumboard panelling. This will also make the workshop a lot more comfortable in winter.

HOUSE PAINT KEEPS PEELING

Within a year after it is applied, paint begins to peel off our wood siding, so I have to repaint the house every two years. It is 30 years old and the paint stayed on fine for 10 years. What am I doing wrong?

When paint blisters it usually indicates that moisture is coming through from behind. The most common cause of this, particularly in an older house without a vapor barrier on the inside wall, is too much humidity indoors during cold weather. Water vapor passes through the wall, condenses behind the wood siding and eventually gets under the paint. You may find, for instance, that the blistering is worse outside of rooms where moisture originates, such as the bathroom, but it can occur wherever humidity is high enough to cause dripping windows and damp walls. The remedy is to provide more ventilation during cold weather. Just watch your windows; when they stop steaming up you have enough.

Another factor may be too many coats of paint. I estimate that there are at least 10 coats of paint on the siding, and some of the earlier coats may be pulling away from the wood by now. It may be time to have all the paint stipped off and start again. I recommend using latex primer and paint next time; water-based paints are more resistant to blistering than alkyd or other solvent-thinned finishes.

PAINT PEELING AROUND CEILING FIXTURE

We want to redecorate our bedrooms, but don't know what to do about the paint that keeps peeling off the ceiling around the light fixtures. That's the only place this problem occurs. What would be causing this?

It's probably due to condensation inside the ceiling hole. A lot of warm, humid household air leaks through this into the cold attic during the winter. Most hardware stores sell circular pads of a plastic foam material that can be inserted between the base of the light fixture and the ceiling to prevent air leakage.

POWDERY FILM ON PAINT

The plywood soffits under the overhang of my roof are painted with latex in a dark accent color. A whitish powder has appeared on this in some areas. The oil-based paint that was on before was also covered with this powdery film. What causes this and what can I do about it?

All exterior paints break down slowly on exposure to the weather, producing a chalky surface that normally washes away with the rain, an action that actually makes the paint self-cleaning. But because the soffit is sheltered from the rain, the chalk dust builds up, and must be washed off before the surface can be repainted. Use a stiff brush and a solution of ¼ cup of trisodium phosphate (TSP) to a gallon of water.

NON-TOXIC PAINT

We are expecting our second child and would like to repaint the crib, but we have been unable to find a paint that is specifically labelled as being non-toxic.

For some years now, product safety regulations have required that all paints sold for interior use in homes be non-toxic. A high-gloss enamel would be easiest to keep clean.

PAINT REMOVING

PAINT REMOVER RECIPE

I have just bought an old table that is covered with many coats of paint, but I suspect there may be some nice wood underneath. Someone told me that lye would be a good paint remover to use on something like this. Can you tell me how to mix and use this?

In an 8-ounce glass jar, dissolve two heaping tablespoons of lye in four ounces of cold water. In another jar the same size, stir one level tablespoon of cornstarch in half a cup of cold water, then add this to the lye solution while stirring. It will thicken to a paste-like consistency almost immediately.

Take the table outside and brush this paste on the paint with an old nylon paint brush. Wear rubber gloves and be careful to keep the lye solution off everything but the paint, which will be soft enough to remove with a putty knife in from 30 to 60 minutes, depending on the temperature. More than one application may be necessary to remove several coats of paint, but as soon as you get down to the wood, wash the lye solution off thoroughly to keep it from softening the wood.

This work should only be done outdoors or in a basement with an unfinished concrete floor and good drainage. Unused lye solution can be stored in a covered jar. (It also makes a good oven cleaner.)

REMOVING PAINT FROM ARBORITE

When I was painting our kitchen cupboards I spilled some on the Arborite countertop. I thought I had wiped it up, but now I see there are some spots that I missed. How can I remove these without harming the countertop?

The protective layer of melamine plastic used on Arborite and Formica is unaffected by ordinary paint removers. Use one of these to soften the paint, then wipe it off with a nylon scouring pad.

REMOVER FOR MILK PAINT

We moved into an older home some months ago and decided to clean up the coal-burning fireplace. In the process we discovered that what appeared to be brown tiles around the face of the fireplace were actually lovely blue ceramic tiles that had been painted. A lot of work with a paint remover had taken all of this off except for a coat of some kind of white paint that is not affected by the paint remover. What can I use to take this off?

If ordinary paint removers won't touch it, this may be an old-fashioned casein paint or milk paint. A strong ammonia solution should take this off.

REMOVING PAINT FROM MORTAR

The previous owner of our house applied black paint to the mortar joints in an otherwise lovely stone fireplace in our living room. Is there anything that will remove the paint from the mortar without damaging it? If not, can I apply a thin layer of plain mortar over the paint?

Ordinary paint remover will soften the paint so it can be scrubbed off with a stiff brush, but mortar is quite porous and you may not be able to remove it all. A thin layer of new mortar will not stick to the paint; you would have to remove it at least half an inch deep in order to apply new mortar. I think the best remedy is to cover the black paint with two coats of a flat latex paint in the color you want.

REMOVING PEELING PAINT

The paint on the wood siding of our house has peeled and cracked very badly. What is the best way to prepare this for repainting? Do I have to remove all the old paint?

If this is an old house with many layers of paint, it would be best to strip them all off and start again. I would use an electric hot air gun for this job. But if the peeling paint does not appear to be very thick, or does not cover too large an area, I would be inclined just to scrape off the loose paint with a broad putty knife and then taper the remaining edges with sandpaper so they will not show through the new finish. Round the edges of the putty knife with a file to keep them from digging into the wood. Apply a coat of primer to the exposed wood before repainting.

REMOVING PAINT FROM VINYL SIDING

When I was painting our eavestroughs and soffits I spilled a little paint on the vinyl siding. Now it has hardened and I don't know how to take it off without damaging the siding.

If you test in some inconspicuous spot, I think you will find that the vinyl siding is unaffected by regular paint remover, available at any hardware store.

PAINTING

PAINTING ALUMINUM SIDING

The white aluminum siding on our house has become quite dirty over the years and is difficult to clean. We think a darker color would look better and would like to know if the siding can be painted.

Aluminum siding can be painted, but it will not last as long as the original factory finish. It should be good for about five years, however. The first step is a thorough cleaning to remove mildew, dirt and chalked paint. Use a solution of one part chlorine laundry bleach (liquid) to three parts water, plus half a cup of *dishwasher* detergent per gallon (or 30ml per litre). Apply with a stiff brush and rinse thoroughly with a hose. Allow to dry before painting.

A flat paint will do the best job of hiding small irregularities in the thin metal, such as minor dents or ripples. Even a semi-gloss finish can make these more apparent. An exterior acrylic latex paint is recommended. (Most alkyd or "oil-based" house paints have too much sheen for this application.) This can be applied directly to the siding after it has been cleaned, but for better adhesion most paint chemists advise applying an *alkyd* primer first.

PAINTING ASBESTOS SHINGLES

I recently purchased a house that has asbestos shingles on the outside walls. They are in good condition but appear to have been painted previously, and I would like to repaint them. What kind of paint should I use? Is a primer necessary? Are there any special precautions I should take because of the asbestos in them?

Such shingles are made of portland cement (as in concrete) reinforced with a small amount of asbestos fibres. Since these are entirely enclosed in the rigid cement they do not present any health hazard and require no special preparation or precautions when painting them. Simply remove any loose paint with a stiff brush, then apply an exterior latex house paint.

PAINTING A BASEBOARD HEATER

The electric baseboard heater in our bathroom has a number of chips and rust spots on it. We would also like to change the color. Is there a special kind of paint that must be used?

No. The metal jacket of a baseboard heater doesn't get hot enough to require a special, high-temperature paint. Any alkyd enamel will do a good job. Use #120 paper to remove the rust spots and sand down the edges of the chipped areas. If the old finish is glossy, sand the entire surface to remove the shine and provide a "tooth" for the new finish, then apply two coats of enamel to the cold heater and leave the heat off for 48 hours.

PAINTING A BASEMENT FLOOR

Is it necessary to treat the concrete floor in our basement with anything before we paint it? What kind of paint is best?

The floor must be clean and free of oil stains of any kind. These can be removed by wetting the spot and sprinkling it with trisodium phosphate crystals (TSP, available from any hardware store). Brush these in, let stand 15 minutes, then brush again and hose off. Although it is not essential, it is a good idea to etch the concrete with a solution of muriatic acid before painting it. One test that has been suggested is to sprinkle a few drops of water on the dry concrete; if they are not absorbed within five minutes, acid-etching is recommended.

Use one part muriatic acid to 10 parts water. Pour this directly on a clean *wet* floor, spread it with a wide brush and let it stand until it stops foaming, then rinse thoroughly with plain water. It is best to work on an area about 4 square feet at a time. *Do not let the surface dry between etching and rinsing.* Use a mop to remove surface water.

Latex, alkyd and polyurethane concrete floor paints are now available. Alkyd and polyurethane generally wear better than latex and have a higher gloss, but they are also more slippery.

REFINISHING A BATHTUB

We have a lovely old cast iron bathtub that was built into the house. It has been refinished professionally a couple of times (at a cost of $200 each time) but the new enamel didn't last very long. Because of the way the tub is installed we would have to wreck the entire bathroom and remove everything in it to take out the tub. Is there any other way we can refinish it?

You can refinish it yourself with a 2-part epoxy paint such as Klenk's Epoxy Tile & Tub Finish (Swing Paints Limited, Montreal) or Pratt & Lambert's PALGARD. Use #80 silicon carbide paper to roughen the existing finish and provide a "tooth" for the new finish. Mix and apply as directed.

This won't produce as smooth a finish as a professional spray job, but it should last longer than the work you have had done, and it will certainly be a lot cheaper. Epoxy paints are tricky to use, however, because they begin to set as soon as the two parts are mixed. Prepare only as much as you are going to have time to use (the setting time will be given on the label).

PAINTING A CRIB

I have built a baby crib and would like to find a perfectly safe paint to use on it.

For many years, all paints sold on the retail market have had to meet federal health safety standards that are just as strict as those that apply to the finishes used on factory-made baby cribs. Any consumer paint is safe to use, in other words, but I would choose a urethane enamel because of its toughness and durability.

PAINTING A CRUMBLING CEILING

We have a textured ceiling in our living room that looks very nice but is a problem to paint because the surface crumbles when you touch it, and little pellets of some lightweight material fall to the floor. I'm afraid to use either a brush or a roller on it.

Some spray-on ceiling finishes consist of a plaster base mixed with granules of perlite, an expanded volcanic rock, or beads of polystyrene, an insulation material. Properly mixed and applied, it makes a good textured finish, but it is often very difficult to paint. Spray application works best, but you'll have to call in a professional painter for this. If you want to do it yourself, use a flat latex paint and apply it with a lamb's wool roller. Keep the roller well filled with paint and use it in two crosswise directions in order to cover all the hills and valleys evenly. Some of the pellets will come off on the roller, but they will simply mix with the paint and be reapplied.

PAINTING CERAMIC WALL TILES

I don't like the color of the ceramic wall tiles in my bathroom. Can they be painted?

Any interior enamel can be applied to hard, shiny surfaces like this with reasonable success, but the paint will chip off very easily. There are special primers that will hold paint to difficult surfaces like this, but you may have trouble finding them. Three such products I have used are Easy Surface Prep (The Flood Company), Prime-It 20 (Swing Paints Limited), and XIM Flash Bond (XIM Products Canada Limited). Any alkyd or latex paint can be applied over these primers.

PAINTING CHRISTMAS LIGHT BULBS

I have 50 or 60 outdoor Christmas light bulbs that have lost a lot of their color over the years. Can you tell me how to repaint them?

Any paint or enamel can be used. Clean the glass thoroughly first to remove all finger marks, and be careful not to touch the glass afterwards. Use a small, flat brush to apply the paint. Put an elastic band around the base and use an unbent paper clip as a hook to hang the bulb from a line until the paint dries. One coat should be enough.

PAINTING A FRIDGE

We are remodeling our kitchen and replacing some of the appliances, but would like to keep our present fridge. Unfortunately it does not match the new color scheme. Is there any place we can have it repainted?

Any auto paint shop could do it for you, I'm sure. They are experts at matching colors and the finish should be as good as the original. You can paint it yourself, however, if you can find the color you want among the hundreds of tones that are now available at paint and hardware stores. Rub the present finish with #00 steel wool to remove the gloss and provide a "tooth" for the new finish, preferably a gloss or semi-gloss enamel.

PAINTING AN ELECTRIC STOVE

You have given advice on repainting a refrigerator to match a new stove and dishwasher. My problem is the other way around; I would like to repaint our electric stove to match other new appliances.

A heat resistant paint would be needed to withstand the high temperature around the surface elements and the oven door. Such paints can be found at auto supply stores but the color range is very limited and you are not likely to find a match for your other appliances. It is doubtful, too, if such a paint would adhere well to the high-temperature, porcelainized finish used on a stove. In short, I don't think it is a good idea.

PAINTING A MAHOGANY DOOR

The doors inside my house are faced with mahogany plywood that has been given a dark stain. I would like to paint them to match the walls. Does mahogany need any special preparation for painting?

Philippine mahogany is an open-grained wood with a very porous surface. For a smooth finish, the open pores should be filled before painting. Ask your paint or hardware store for a "wood finishing filler". Thin it to a brushing consistency and then apply to about a quarter of the door panel. After not more than five minutes, wipe the filler off across the grain with a pad of burlap or other coarse cloth, or scrape it off with a broad putty knife or a piece of cardboard, then wipe clean. The object is to leave the filler in the grain pores but remove it from the surface. Do the remainder of the door the same

way, one manageable area at a time, being careful not to let the filler dry too much before you wipe or scrape it off. After 24 hours, sand lightly and apply your primer and finish coats as required.

PAINTING OVER VARNISH

All the interior doors in our house have a clear varnish finish. We would like to paint them to match the walls and wood trim. Is there a special primer or other treatment that must be applied to the varnish so it will accept the paint, or must we remove it all?

All you have to do is sandpaper the varnish lightly to remove the gloss and provide a better bonding surface for the paint. No primer is required but you will probably need two coats of paint.

PAINTING PARTICLE BOARD

I have made a few things out of particle board, but when I paint this it shows a textured surface like orange skin. How can I get a smoother finish?

Apply an alkyd primer, sand lightly, remove the sanding dust and then fill the textured surface with spackling compound (DAP is one brand) or a premixed crack-filler such as Polyfix. Apply this with a broad putty knife, then smooth with fine sandpaper on a wood block. Finish with two coats of alkyd enamel.

PAINTING RADIATORS

We have an older home with hot water heating and cast iron radiators. There are many coats of paint on these radiators and we think we could reduce our heating bills a lot if we remove all the paint. How can we do this? What is the best color to use? We have noticed that radiators in public buildings are often painted silver. Does this get more heat out of the radiators?

The number of coats of paint makes no noticeable difference in the amount of heat that is given off by a radiator; paint has virtually no insulation value at all. The color does not make much difference, either. While it is true that a flat black surface radiates heat fractionally better that a glossy white surface, the difference between any two house paints would not be detectable. And even if there was a difference, this would not mean that you would lose or gain heat. A slight reduction in the amount of heat given off by a radiator would merely increase the temperature of the circulating water, and so the heat would still be distributed to the house.

The paint can be removed, however, with any of the commercial paint removers. Several applications will be needed to take off all the layers. But don't do this while the radiators are hot; wait until the heating system is shut down.

The silver paint you see on some radiators is simply aluminum paint. This looks nice in some situations, but it will not improve heat output. The paint you use on your walls is the best one to use on the radiators.

PAINTING SOFFITS

I have tried for several years to paint the plywood soffits under our roof overhang, but the paint keeps peeling off. Can you tell me why it is doing this?

Water could be backing up behind an ice dam and running under the shingles into the overhang, but more likely the paint is peeling because you are not removing the chalky surface of the paint before repainting. All house paints turn chalky with age, but this is normally removed by the rain – a self-cleaning action, really. Protected surfaces such as roof overhangs and porch ceilings never get cleaned this way, however, so you have to wash them by hand before you paint them. Paint will not adhere to a powdery surface.

PAINTING A SWIMMING POOL

We have an in-ground, poured concrete swimming pool that I have painted every three or four years with epoxy. My trouble is that after a couple of years the paint begins to rub off on your skin when it is touched, and brushing the pool produces clouds of powdered paint. Is there another kind of paint I should use next time? I have noticed some latex house paints advertised as being non-peeling and non-chalking, and they are a lot cheaper than epoxy. Could one of these be used?

A certain amount of chalking is normal, but you should get at least five years service out of an epoxy pool finish, which most experts agree is the best paint for a concrete pool. Not all epoxy paints are suitable for pools, however, and the excessive chalking in your case may be due to using a product that was not designed for this job. Or perhaps you are not mixing enough hardener with the epoxy. Failure to maintain the proper pH level in the water could also contribute to the problem, pool experts tell me.

Latex house paint is not suitable for a pool, but other types of pool paint are available. Chlorinated rubber paint rates close to epoxy in durability, and is the only kind that doesn't get chalky with age. You can also use a latex-modified cement paint (quite different from a latex house paint), or even regular boat hull enamel. But if you switch to another kind of paint you have to have all the epoxy paint removed first with sandblasting.

PAINTING OVER WALLPAPER

We want to paint some gypsumboard walls that have been papered. Is there anything special we have to do to them after we remove the wallpaper?

If the wallpaper is firmly attached, the easiest thing to do is just paint over it with an alkyd or other oil-based paint. This is certainly advisable if the paper was applied with a standard adhesive, which can be very difficult to remove. Modern, pre-pasted, dry-strippable papers usually come off very easily, but the adhesive that is left on the wall will have to be washed off with a solution of one tablespoon of trisodium phosphate (TSP) to a quart of water. Apply with a cloth or sponge but wipe it off quickly to avoid soaking the gypsumboard.

If it is a vinyl-coated wallpaper, however, only the surface layer will peel away, leaving the paper backing on the wall. This will have to be removed before the wall can be painted. The best way to do this is to dampen the paper with a sponge and scrape it off with a broad putty knife or similar tool, then wash the wall with the TSP solution as described above to remove the adhesive.

TEXTURED WALLS

We are remodelling an old house and are trying to decide how to finish the walls, which we have panelled with gypsumboard. Friends of ours have a very attractive recreation room that was done in an Old English style with fake beams and rough plaster walls created with a textured paint. Do you think this would be suitable for the main living area of our house?

If that's the style you want, there's no reason why you can't have it. But once you apply that type of finish you're going to have to live with it for a long time. It is very difficult to remove these heavily textured, plaster-based finishes and restore a smooth surface suitable for painting or papering.

WHITEWASH FORMULA

I have a very long fence around my property that I would like to whitewash. Can you give me a formula to make my own whitewash? I can't afford paint.

Whitewash is not very weatherproof, but it's certainly cheap - you can make it for as little as $1 a gallon. The basic ingredient is lime paste - hydrated lime or calcium hydroxide - which turns to calcium carbonate or chalk on exposure to air. Be sure to get hydrated lime or agricultural "spray lime", not the crushed limestone sold for dressing lawns. It is available at some garden shops and all farm supply stores. The following formula will make about 2½ gallons of whitewash:

Soak 10 pounds of hydrated lime in 1 gallon of water and stir to make a paste. Dissolve 3 pounds of salt in 5 quarts of water and add this to the lime paste. Add water if necessary to make a *thin* paint.

If you prefer metric, soak 3.5 kg of hydrated lime in 3.5 litres of water. Dissolve 1 kg of salt in 4 litres of water and add it to the above mixture. Makes about 9 litres.

PLUMBING

DRAIN GURGLES WHEN TOILET FLUSHED

We recently bought a 12-year-old, 2-storey house. It has a full bathroom and a half bathroom or powder room on the second floor. The problem is that when either of the upstairs toilets is flushed there is a gurgling sound in the bathtub drain. Is this something that should be repaired?

The gurgling sound means that water is being sucked out of the bathtub drain trap, and this could allow sewer gases to enter the house. There must be something wrong with the vent pipe connection to the bathtub drain line. It may be plugged, but my guess is that it's too far from the bathtub drain - the plumbing code requires it to be within 5 ft. Ask a plumber to check this for you and suggest what changes should be made.

DRAINING THE WATER SYSTEM

We are going to leave our house for the winter, and have decided not to keep the heat on. How do we drain the water system to prevent any of the pipes bursting?

It is impossible to drain all of the pipes. The short length of pipe coming into the house behind the main shut-off valve, for instance, cannot be drained, and if this bursts the basement could be flooded. Flooding can be prevented by having the water turned off at the supply main, but this would not prevent the pipe from bursting where it enters the house, and you would have a lot of trouble when the water supply was turned on again. Even some interior pipes cannot be drained properly - up-feed pipes to a water tank or boiler, for instance - and these might have to be replaced before the water service could be restored. It would be a lot safer, and perhaps even cheaper, to leave a little heat on while you are away. And did you know that your insurance requires the house to be inspected regularly by a responsible adult?

FROST IN PLUMBING VENT PIPE

Our country home has a septic tank that works fine except for one annoying problem. The vent pipe that goes up through the roof gets plugged with frost during very cold weather, and allows sewer gases to get into the house. Each time this happens I have to go up on the roof with boiling water to thaw the pipe open, but a few weeks later it is plugged again. How can I cure this problem?

If the vent pipe passes through an attic space you can reach, simply wrap the pipe with batt insulation tied with string. This should keep the rising air in the pipe warm enough to prevent ice forming in the section above the roof. If you cannot reach the vent pipe at that point, you may be able to buy an insulating sleeve that fits over the pipe above the roof. And if you can't find that, you can make your own with a piece of plastic drain pipe about 1½ in. larger in diameter than the vent pipe. Cut the bottom to fit the roof slope and the top to match the height of the vent pipe. Wrap the vent pipe with enough soft polyurethane upholstery foam padding to fill the space between the two pipes. Tape or tie this in place, then slip the larger pipe over it, caulking it around the bottom. Add a cone-shaped rain cap large enough to shelter the sleeve.

HOT WATER PRESSURE LOW

We have lots of pressure in our cold water pipes, but the hot water taps run very slowly, even when fully open. The bathroom sink, tub and shower are the worst. We tried draining some water from the tank, thinking it might be blocked with sludge, but this didn't help. The water in our area isn't as soft as it should be; could this be the cause? If so, what can be done about it?

It is almost certainly due to a buildup of lime deposit in the pipes. This happens much faster in the hot water pipes than in the cold ones, and the bathroom taps are probably used much more than any others in the house.

Unfortunately, the only remedy is to have the pipes replaced. There is no way to remove the lime deposit from the pipes. To prevent the problem from occurring again, it might be advisable to install a water softener.

HOT WATER TAPS SPURT

Amost every time we turn on a hot water tap, hot air and water spurt out. The cold water taps don't do this. Can you tell me what causes this and how to cure it?

A mixture of air and water spurting out of the hot water taps usually indicates that the water temperature is too high. Try lowering the thermostat setting on the water heater. If this does not cure the problem it may be due to gas produced by an overactive magnesium anode in the hot water tank. One remedy for this is to replace the magnesium rod with an aluminium one. These are now available for most water heaters, and any plumber can install one for you.

RUNNING OUT OF HOT WATER

Our gas-fired hot water tank has worked fine for 10 years, but recently it has been running out of water very quickly. There is hardly enough for one bath. What could cause this? The thermostat hasn't been changed.

There could be something wrong with the thermostatic gas valve that controls the water temperature, but more likely the trouble is caused by a corroded dip pipe inside the tank. This takes the incoming cold water to the bottom of the tank. Sometimes it corrodes and breaks off, however, allowing cold water to enter near the top of the tank, where it will mix with the hot water. Your gas company will check these possibilities for you.

NOT ENOUGH HOT WATER

My electric hot water tank still heats up quickly and the water is as hot as ever, but the supply runs out much quicker than it did just a week or so ago. What would cause this?

Probably one of the heating elements is not operating. There are two elements in your water heater, but only one is on at a time. When hot water is drawn from the top of the tank, the element there comes on to heat up more water, but when the water temperature reaches the element's thermostat setting it switches the electric current to the heating element in the bottom of the tank. It sounds as if the element in the bottom of your tank has burned out or its thermostat is not working properly. Have it checked by an electrician.

REMOVING POP-UP DRAIN PLUG

The bathroom sink where I wash my hair isn't draining very well. How do I remove the pop-up stopper to clean the drain?

Some pop-up drain plugs can be removed simply by giving them half a turn to unhook them from the pivot rod at the bottom, then lifting them out. Try turning yours in both directions. If it does not come loose you'll have to remove the pivot rod at the back of the drainpipe under the sink. To do this, you must unscrew the knurled cap that holds the rod in the drainpipe, then pull out the rod and lift up the drain plug. (The knurled cap also tightens or loosens the movement of the drain plug.)

REMOVING A TAP HANDLE

I want to replace the washer in the bathtub tap that's leaking, but the handle is stuck on the stem. I have removed the snap-in cap and the screw underneath that holds the handle on, but it won't budge.

Try a few drops of penetrating oil such as WD40 or Liquid Wrench, then wait an hour or so for the oil to work its way into the frozen joint. Plumbers use a tool called, logically enough, a "handle puller". You can buy one of these at a plumbing supply store if the penetrating oil doesn't work.

REPLACING SINK DRAIN

The chrome-plated ring around the drain of our bathroom sink has chipped and the metal underneath is rusting. Is there any way I can fix this?

There's no way you can re-chrome the drain fitting, but it's not difficult to install a new one. You simply unscrew the trap and tailpiece under the sink, then undo the large nut that holds the drain fitting and push this up into the sink. Take it to a plumbing supply shop for a replacement PO plug, as it is called. Put a bead of plumber's putty under the lip when the new fitting is installed. Fit the rubber washer and nut in place under the sink and tighten the drain fitting, then reconnect the drain trap.

CARE OF A SEPTIC TANK

Would you please give me some information on the care and maintenance of a septic tank? This is our first summer in a new cottage and we are getting a lot of different advice on what household chemicals we can and cannot use, whether additives are necessary to keep the tank working properly, and how often it needs to be cleaned.

A septic tank built and installed to present standards will not be harmed by any common household chemical used in reasonable amounts. That includes acids, alkalis, detergents, toilet bowl cleaners, drain cleaners, bleach, lye, permanent wave solutions, cosmetics, bath oils and water softeners. Government experts also say that none of the so-called "activators" are needed to keep a septic tank operating properly. Organic wastes are broken down by a perfectly natural bacterial action, and everything that is necessary, including the bacteria, is amply provided by the waste materials themselves. Insoluable materials settle to the bottom of the tank, however, and have to be removed periodically. A septic tank should be inspected once a year, but normally will only have to be pumped out about every three years. There are companies in all rural areas that do this work quickly, cleanly and efficiently.

GARBAGE DISPOSAL UNIT vs SEPTIC TANK

Our house has a septic tank system, and my husband maintains that this will not permit us to install a garbage disposal unit in the kitchen sink. A friend, however, says that **this will actually improve the operation of the septic tank. Please tell me whether or not we can have a garbage disposal unit installed?**

Garbage is, indeed, food for the bacteria that break down the organic waste in a septic tank. The only problem is the capacity of the tank. If it was installed in recent years it is probably big enough to handle the extra load without any trouble. But even if it is a small tank put in many years ago, adding a garbage disposal unit would only mean that you will have to have the tank checked and cleaned more often. Whether or not it's worth the extra trouble and expense is up to you.

SHOWER PRESSURE LOW

I installed a shower using ½ in. copper pipe, and now it is the only water fixture in the house that has insufficient pressure. What did I do wrong?

If you cut the pipe with a tube cutter that clamps on the pipe and uses a small blade wheel to score it, you may have forgotten to remove the burr inside the pipe with the reamer attached to the cutter. The burr left by the cutter can reduce the effective diameter of the pipe enough to restrict the water flow.

WHY DOES THE SHOWER TEMPERATURE CHANGE?

Can you explain why the temperature in my bathroom shower changes whenever someone turns on a tap somewhere else in the house? I can understand a drop in *pressure* when the water is being used elsewhere, but I don't see why the temperature should change. I'm tired of getting alternately frozen and scalded. Is there any way to prevent this?

It is the change in pressure that causes the change in temperature. When a cold or hot water tap is turned on anywhere else in the house it causes a drop in pressure *in that line only*. If it is a cold tap, the cold water pressure drops in your shower and the spray mixture gets hotter. (The shower pressure also drops slightly, of course, but you don't notice this.) Conversely, if someone turns on a hot water tap, the pressure in that line drops and your shower turns cold.

To overcome this problem, plumbing manufacturers have developed a "pressure balancing valve" for bathroom showers. When the water pressure drops in either the hot or cold supply line the pressure on the other line is automatically adjusted so the mixture balance stays the same. (But the temperature will still drop if you run out of hot water, of course.) Any plumbing supply store can show you the models that are available, and any plumber can install one. I don't recommend it as a do-it-yourself job.

SINK BACKS UP

I live on the first floor of an apartment building, and would like to know why soapy water somtimes comes gushing up in my sink. There is a laundry room on this floor. Do you think it could come from there?

Excessive use of laundry detergents can cause a temporary blockage in the drain, particularly if it has not been designed too well. This could cause a backflow into your sink when an overhead drain was used. It's not a very pleasant prospect and your landlord should certainly fix it. Report the problem to him in writing and keep a copy for youself. It may only require cleaning out the drain lines, but that's not something that you can do.

SINK DRAIN GURGLES

I recently replaced the drain line from our kitchen sink to the basement. Since then the sink works fine except for a gurgling sound it makes when the last of the water drains away. What would cause this?

Most likely you haven't connected the vent pipe correctly. Every sink, tub and other plumbing fixture is fitted with a U-shaped trap behind the drain. Enough water must remain in this at all times to prevent sewer gases from coming back into the house through the drain openings. To keep the trap from being syphoned dry when the sink is drained, an air vent pipe that extends up through the roof must be connected to the drain line within 5 ft of the trap.

The gurgling sound you hear is the sink trap being syphoned dry because the vent pipe is missing, plugged, or incorrectly connected. You can find out if it is plugged by going up on the roof and putting a garden hose in the vent pipe. If the water backs up, the pipe is plugged. Usually the force of the water will clear it, however. If the pipe is not plugged, the simplest remedy would be to add an automatic plumbing vent to the drain pipe just behind the sink trap. These are available at all plumbing stores.

SLOW SINK

Ever since we started using it, the bathroom sink in our new home has drained very slowly. Then, just as the sink is emptying, a big bubble comes out of the drain and the rest of the water rushes away freely. The builder sent the plumber around but he said he couldn't find anything wrong. Obviously the drain isn't plugged. Do you know what's causing this annoying problem?

I think the trouble is in the strainer that you can see when you look down the sink drain. Sometimes the crossbars in the strainer are too large, making the drain holes so small that an air bubble is trapped underneath them and prevents the water flowing freely. You can test this by pushing a soda straw down through the strainer when the sink is draining slowly. This will release the air bubble and allow the water to drain away normally.

One remedy is to enlarge the openings between the crossbars of the strainer with a triangular file. Another is to replace the tailpipe and strainer in the sink. Unscrew the locknut under the sink, push up the tailpipe and remove the strainer ring from the sink. Replace with one with larger openings.

SOLDERING COPPER PIPE

I've been practicing soldering copper pipes and fittings with a view to doing some minor plumbing modifications in my basement. I find I can do a neat job with the actual soldering, but have trouble getting an even coat of solder on the pipe first, an operation that is called "tinning", I believe. I usually end up with a blob of solder on the bottom of the pipe. Is tinning really necessary?

Tinning isn't necessary if both surfaces have been rubbed down to bare, shiny metal with steel wool before the flux is applied. Another trick that helps to draw the molten solder into the joint is to apply the torch to the larger part, about an inch *behind* the edge. Solder always flows towards the heat.

TOILET DOESN'T FLUSH PROPERLY

Our toilet doesn't flush properly. We have to hold the handle down all the time it's flushing, otherwise it stops. How can we fix this?

The chain that lifts the plug out of the bottom of the toilet tank is too long. This should be just long enough to let the plug drop in the opening when the handle is up. You can shorten it by moving the chain up a few links. Some toilets use a lift wire instead of a chain. This can be shortened by bending the upper wire.

TOILET NOT FLUSHING PROPERLY

The toilet in our basement does not flush properly; sometimes even a Kleenex tissue will not flush away. A plumber removed the toilet to check the drain, but found nothing wrong. The problem is still there; could it be in the toilet itself?

If the drain is clear the problem must be in the toilet. Remove the lid from the water tank to see if it is filling and emptying properly. If the water level does not come up to the mark on the tank (usually about 2 ½ in. below the rim), bend or otherwise adjust the float arm up until the water level is correct. On the other hand, if the tank is not emptying completely, the flap or ball valve in the bottom of the tank must be closing too quickly. Shorten the chain or wire that connects the valve to the flusing lever.

If the water level is not the problem, you probably have a jet-action toilet that uses a strong jet of water entering the back of the bowl to start the syphon action that empties it. The jet hole sometimes gets plugged with lime buildup, but can be cleared quite easily with a length of coathanger wire.

RUSTY GEL IN TOILET TANK

When I had to adjust the float arm in my toilet tank recently I noticed a rust-brown, jelly-like coating on the tank and the fittings inside it. What causes this and how can I prevent it?

This not uncommon condition is caused by a type of bacteria that actually live on, and consume, iron, forming a rust-colored, gelatinous deposit on the metal and other surfaces. Turn off the water supply to the tank and flush it empty, then use a scrubbing brush and a solution of powdered floor cleaner or dishwasher detergent to remove the deposit. Refill and flush the tank to clean it out. As it refills again, add a quart of chlorine laundry bleach. Let this stand for several hours before flushing to sterilize the tank. Adding a couple of cups of bleach to the tank once a month or so will prevent the iron bacteria from becoming established again.

TOILET BOWL DOESN'T REFILL

Our toilet bowl doesn't refill properly after it's flushed. The water only comes up about half way. Can you tell me what's causing this and what I can do about it?

There is probably something wrong with the refill tube inside the water tank. This is a small rubber tube that comes off the side of the ballcock valve at the end of the float arm. The other end of the refill tube goes in the top of the 1 in. diameter overflow pipe that stands in the middle of the tank. Perhaps the refill tube has slipped out of the overflow pipe (it's usually held there by a bent wire clip). Or the tube may be plugged with lime deposit. In the latter case, either clear the tube or replace it.

TOILET TANK DOESN'T FILL

Can you tell me what controls the level of the water in a toilet tank? Ours does not fill as high as it used to.

The water level is controlled by a float, usually a ball at one end of a hinged lever. The refilling valve (called a ballcock valve) is located at the other end of the lever, at the top of the water supply pipe. The correct water level is marked on the inside of the tank, but is usually about half an inch below the top of the open overflow pipe in the centre of the tank. If the level is much lower than that, there are two possible causes. The float may have water in it, in which case it should be replaced. Or the float arm may be bent downwards, causing it to shut the water off too soon. The simple remedy for that is to bend the float arm up as much as you want to raise the level of the water.

The other possibility is that the stopper or flap valve at the bottom of the tank is not closing properly, either because it is damaged or the valve seat is dirty. (If this is the cause, however, you would hear water running constantly.) The remedy is to replace the damaged valve or wipe the valve seat clean.

LIME IN TOILET TANK

Our water is very hard and a buildup of lime in the toilet tank is preventing the toilet from flushing properly. How can we remove this?

Pour a cupful of muriatic acid in the toilet tank and let it stand until the lime deposit stops bubbling. If some lime remains, add more acid.

SELF-STARTING TOILET

We have a toilet with a very strange problem. Once every hour or so it flushes all by itself. When I rush in to see what is happening, the water is just rising the last inch or so in the tank and the water in the bowl seems undisturbed. A plumber I spoke to doesn't believe me. Can you solve the mystery?

I had heard of this problem before and could not believe it either until a neighbor told me he was having the same trouble and I went to have a look at it. It turns out that it is not the toilet *flushing* that you hear, but the sound of the tank *filling*, and only a few inches at that. What is happening is that the flap valve at the bottom of the toilet tank is leaking, and the water runs silently into the bowl. But as the water level in the tank drops, the float valve opens suddenly and refills the tank, and this is a sound many people associate with the flushing action.

The problem may be caused simply by some dirt on the flap valve. Turn off the water supply to the toilet and then flush it to empty the tank. Lift the flap valve and wipe it and the valve seat with a wet cloth to remove any dirt particles that may be holding it open. Open the supply valve to refill the tank. If this does not correct the problem, replace the flap valve with a new one available at any hardware or plumbing supply store.

TOILET TANK VIBRATES

When our toilet refills there is a loud vibrating noise that seems to come from the tank. I can stop the noise by turning on the cold water tap in the bathtub, so I assume it is a venting problem.

Venting problems only occur in drain lines. This is a supply line problem and it is probably caused by a loose ballcock valve inside the tank – the filling valve, in other words. High water pressure is a contributing factor, however, and this is why turning on the bathtub tap will correct it. A simple remedy would be to close the supply line valve under the tank slightly, but then the tank would take longer to fill.

A better remedy is to repair the loose valve, which is not difficult to do. First pick up a ballcock repair kit from your hardware store for two or three dollars. Turn off the water supply to the toilet tank and flush the toilet to empty it, then remove the float arm and lift out the ballcock plunger. If the washer on the bottom is loose, simply tightening the screw may cure your problem, but it is better to put in a new washer from your kit. The ring gasket around the plunger should also be replaced. Reassemble the ballcock valve and float arm and turn on the water.

FIXING A MODERN TOILET VALVE

You have told how to replace the washer in a toilet tank filler valve to stop it leaking or vibrating. You described the traditional kind with a brass plunger that is operated by the float arm and has a washer on the bottom. I have one of the modern filler valves that is made of white plastic with the float arm permanently attached to it. There is a large rubber disc inside the top, but no washer that I can see. How can I stop this from leaking?

This is a diaphragm-type water control valve, and you can buy a replacement kit for it in a plumbing store if you give them the name of the model you have. This is stamped on the top of the valve assembly. There are several different types of diaphragm valves, and the parts look very similar, so it is a good idea to take the old rubber disc to the store with you so you can be sure of getting the replacement kit you need.

TREE ROOTS IN SEWER PIPE

Our main sewer pipe was clogged with roots from three large poplar trees in our back yard. This has been cleared now, but I'm afraid the roots will grow back. If we have the trees cut down, will the roots keep growing?

Sucker shoots will come up and some root growth will continue unless you kill the tree by drilling 3/4 in. holes in the top of the stump and filling them with one of the systemic weed killers such as 2-4-D. If you don't want to remove the trees you can root prune them by digging a deep trench about halfway between the trees and the drain pipe and cutting all roots you encounter.

Both of these jobs will involve a lot of work, however, and it might be better to have the drain pipe replaced. It is probably an old cast iron pipe with bell joints where the packing has cracked. The roots will have opened these cracks, allowing sewage to leak out. I suggest you get some bids on these jobs to help you decide which remedy to undertake.

TUB TAP LEAKS WHEN SHOWER USED

When I turn the handle that switches the water from the bathtub to the showerhead, water still runs out of the tub tap and the flow from the shower is weak. It didn't do this before.

You probably need a new O-ring in the shower diverter valve, the one that switches the water from the tub to the shower. To repair this you have to take out the valve stem. With both taps turned off, remove the diverter handle and the escutcheon plate behind it, if there is one. You will now be able to see either one brass nut at the base of the valve stem, or two, a small nut in front and a larger one behind it.

If you can only see one nut, and it is too far inside the wall to get a crescent wrench on it, measure the size of the nut with the tips of a pair of scissors and then buy a faucet socket wrench of this size from a plumbing supply store. Use the wrench to remove the diverter valve so you can replace the rubber O-rings on the end of it.

But if you can see two brass nuts at the base of the valve stem, *remove only the large one,* as described above. The small one is just a packing nut, but it also reinforces the larger bonnet nut so the soft brass shell won't bend when a wrench is applied.

TUB/SHOWER VALVE DOESN'T WORK

When I lift the button on the bathtub spout to divert water to the shower head, a stream of water still runs from the tub spout. How can I fix this?

There is something wrong with the diverter in the tub spout. The simplest remedy is to unscrew the spout and replace it with a new one. Push a piece of wood or a metal rod up the spout and use this as a lever to turn the spout anti-clockwise. Brush the threads with pipe joint compound before screwing on the new spout.

WATER HEATER KEEPS SHUTTING OFF

Our 40-gallon electric hot water tank has worked well for about 15 years, but now it shuts off every few days and we have to keep pushing the reset button behind the thermostat panel. Why does this happen?

The reset button is a safety switch that turns off the power to the heating element when the water in the tank gets too hot. It is usually set for 180°F (82°C). The most likely explanation is that one of the thermostats that control the two heating elements has welded in the ON position, causing the water to overheat. Since you say it takes a few days for this to happen, it's probably the bottom element, which has a lower wattage than the upper one in water heaters manufactured when yours was. The faulty thermostat will have to be replaced, but it may be better to get a new tank. This one is not going to last much longer.

WATER SOFTENER vs SEPTIC TANK

In our country home we have a water softener that backwashes twice a week into the laundry tub and then into the septic tank. Is the salt solution harmful to the septic tank or the disposal field?

A provincial booklet on the operation of septic tank disposal systems says: "Waste discharges from a household water softener appear to have no adverse effect on the action of a septic tank, but may cause slight shortening of the life of a tile field installed in certain (unspecified) clay soils".

WATER TANK VALVE LEAKS

The temperature/pressure relief valve on my gas-fired water heater was leaking and I replaced it with a new valve about three months ago, but this did not correct the problem. The water temperature and pressure at the taps seems normal. What else could cause the relief valve to leak?

The simplest explanation is that a little bit of dirt is stuck under the sealing disc in the valve. Opening and closing it a few times with the manual lever will sometimes correct this. There is another possibility, however. When cold water enters the tank and is heated, it expands. If there is something that prevents the water from moving backwards in the pipe to accommodate the expansion, and all the taps in your house are closed, then the water can only escape through the pressure relief valve on your heater. The barrier could be an anti-backflow valve in your water supply line, required in some areas, or even a pressure reducing valve that was installed in your house because the pressure in the mains is too high. This is not a serious problem, in any case, and I would simply put a pan under the overflow pipe on the water heater.

WHY NO OVERFLOW OUTLETS IN KITCHEN SINKS?

Someone in our house went out recently and left the water running in the kitchen sink with the stopper closed. The overflow caused a lot of damage. Why are there no overflow outlets in kitchen sinks like there are in bathroom sinks?

That's a very interesting question, and I took it to some of the leading manufacturers of plumbing fixtures. Several could only suggest:

"Because they've always been made that way". But the real answer seems to be that water in a kitchen sink often contains small pieces of vegetables, meat and other organic matter that could lodge inside the overflow pipe and produce a very unpleasant smell, as well as provide a place for the growth of mold and bacteria. Many hospitals, I was told, now require *all* existing sink overflow outlets to be plugged to prevent this, and the new lavatory basins they buy don't have any.

Actually, twin kitchen sinks do have a type of overflow protection. The partition between the two sinks is usually slightly lower than the outside rim, so as long as one drain is open an overflow outlet is available. The sinks must be perfectly level for this to work, however.

ROOFS

CLEANING ASPHALT SHINGLES

We are buying a 10-year-old house with a light grey asphalt shingle roof that looks very dirty and has dark streaks on it. Is there any way we can clean this roof?

I've never heard of anyone cleaning an asphalt shingle roof, and neither has any of the manufacturers I have contacted, but I can see that it might be desirable in some cases. If I wanted to do it I would spray the following solution on the roof with a pump-type, hand-held, garden spray tank: One part chlorine laundry bleach to three parts water, plus one-third of a cup of *dishwasher* detergent per gallon.

To avoid streaks, start at the bottom of the roof and work up. Allow the solution to soak in for 15 minutes or so, then rinse it off with a garden hose. Choose a cloudy day so the solution will not evaporate too quickly. Wetting the roof first might also help. Do not attempt to brush or scrub the dirt off the shingles; this would take off some of the colored granules and allow the sunlight to degrade the asphalt.

CURLING SHINGLES

We had a new asphalt shingle roof put on our garage just three years ago, and already the shingles have started to curl up at the edges. The roofer tells me this is caused by something that is dripping from the leaves of a nearby birch tree. Is there a protective coating of some kind I can paint on the roof?

Your roofer has a great imagination, but his excuse is preposterous. The curling is almost certainly due to the use of defective shingles that were not properly saturated with asphalt. Most likely the roofer obtained factory rejects or "seconds" that are not covered by a warranty and are meant only for use on barns and similar buildings. It may be possible to hold the curled shingles down with dabs of roofing cement or hot melt glue, but the proper remedy is to replace them.

SHINGLES CURLED

We have bought a house that was reshingled a couple of years ago. The asphalt shingles seem to be in good condition except that the tabs on a lot of them are curled up. I tried gluing them down with roofing cement, but this hasn't held very well. What else can I do?

Use a hot-melt glue gun and a long extension cord. Available at any hardware store, these glue guns are fed with sticks or pellets of a thermoplastic ashesive that is squeezed out of the nozzle as a liquid and sets hard in less than a minute. Put a couple of dabs under each tab, then press it down firmly.

REPAIRING EAVESTROUGHS

There is a hole in our galvanized eavestrough that is dripping on our porch, directly in front of the entrance door. What is the best way to fix this?

If the eavestrough is badly corroded, the best remedy is to replace it. Patching is only a temporary cure, but it is easy enough to do with the materials that are now available. Clean the area well and use a wire brush to remove all the rust down to bare metal. Small holes can be filled with a dab of fibrated asphalt roof cement and covered with a piece of aluminum foil to protect the asphalt from sunlight, which degrades it. Or you can buy a small roll of two-inch (50mm) asphalt patching tape backed with aluminum foil. Just cut a piece of this to fit over the hole and press it firmly in place.

If other areas are rusting but not yet leaking, it would be a good idea to remove all the rust from the inside of the eavestrough and then brush on a combined asphalt/aluminum roof coating, available at most hardware and building supply stores. If the outside of the eavestrough also needs painting, use a wire brush to remove all loose paint, clean the bare metal with a cloth soaked in lacquer thinner (much better for this job than petroleum solvent), then apply an alkyd primer and an alkyd exterior trim paint.

PLASTIC EAVESTROUGH CRACKED

Last June I installed plastic eavestroughs on my cottage roof, cementing all the joints as instructed. Recently I noticed that the outside corners have split in the centre of the angle. I have obtained replacement corners but could use some advice on how to install them so they won't crack again.

Vinyl expands and contracts with changes in temperature more than metal does, and if the eavestrough extends around the corners of a roof, as yours does, the instructions call for the use of a special expansion joint that allows the trough section to move. Apparently this wasn't done. Before applying the new corners, install an expansion joint connector in the trough section anywhere between the corners.

FLAT ROOFING

I have a flat roof on my summer cottage that I covered with mineral-surfaced roll roofing a couple of years ago. This has now wrinkled and curled badly and allows water to get underneath, which is going to rot the roof sheathing, of course. How can I repair this?

Mineral-surfaced roll roofing requires a pitch of at least 1:6, and should not be used on a flat roof. What you need is a built-up roof membrane made of several overlapping layers of 15-pound roofing felt bonded with asphalt and topped with gravel. You may not be able to find a roofer to do this in cottage country, but manufacturers such as Domtar, Bakelite and Canadian Gypsum produce cold asphalt roofing adhesives that allow you to do the job yourself. Ask for application instructions.

REPAIRING A FLAT ROOF

Our house has a flat roof about 10 years old coated with tar or asphalt and covered with gravel. There are several places where the tar is exposed, amounting to about 5% of the roof area. Should these be covered with gravel? How long can I expect this type of roof to last? What is the correct way to resurface it?

The gravel is there to protect the bitumen from sunlight that causes it to dry out, crack and become powdery. You should add more gravel to your roof.

Ten to 20 years is the average life of a built-up roof like this. To resurface it, remove the gravel and apply a new 3-ply membrane of 15 lb roofing "felt" (actually paper) layered with hot tar or asphalt. If you want to do the job yourself, use the cold application materials made by Bakelite, Domtar or Canadian Gypsum.

BUILDING A ROOF/SUNDECK

I would like to build a garage with a flat roof that can be used as a sundeck. What kind of roofing should be used?

I know of no roofing material that will withstand regular use as a patio or sundeck. The most practical way to build a usable deck area like this on top of the garage is to put on a conventional built-up, tar-and-gravel roof with good drainage and then add a wood deck built in 4 ft x 4 ft sections that can be removed whenever roof repairs are necessary. Pressure-treated lumber should be used.

SHINGLE GRADES

Our home was built in 1965 and the original asphalt shingles are beginning to show their age. We are thinking of having the roof redone with cedar shakes or shingles, but before deciding we would like to have some information about the different grades that are available in both cedar and asphalt roofing.

Wood seems to be getting more popular for roofing these days, but it is still more expensive than asphalt shingles. Traditional, deeply-ridged cedar shakes are more expensive than taper-sawn cedar shingles, of course, because they use more wood and involve a lot of handwork. Some are still made almost entirely by hand. Most expensive are straight-split shakes, followed by tapersplit, then a type of shake known as handsplit-and-resawn, which is a sort of half shake, half shingle. They all come in only one grade.

Two grades of taper-sawn cedar shingles are acceptable for residential roofing under the National Building Code: No. 1 (blue label) and No. 2 (red label). No. 3 (black label) is recommended only for secondary buildings. To make the question of grades and prices more confusing, all three grades are available in three lengths: 400mm (16 in.), 450mm (18 in.) and 600mm (24 in.).

Until metric measures were introduced, asphalt shingles were graded by the weight of 100 square feet of applied shingles. The lightest grade for residential roofing was 210-pound. For a stronger, more durable roof, 225-pound shingles were available, and some special shingles were graded as 235-pound. Some roofers still refer to these weights, but under metric measure this meaningful terminology has been replaced by two rather vague grades: 10-year warranty and 15-year warranty, the old 210-pound grade now being classed as a 10-year shingle and the other two weights as 15-year shingles.

The warranties only apply to the purchase price of the asphalt shingles if the roof leaks "due to a manufacturing defect", and it is the manufacturer who will decide that. Curling, blisters and loss of granules are not covered, although a manufacturer will sometimes agree to make a contribution to the repair of such a problem. The warranty value also decreases proportionately each month after the first year until the end of the coverage period. But even though these warranties are very limited, all shingle manufacturers provide them and you should insist on getting one from your roofer whenever you have a new roof put on. It gives you the name of the manufacturer, for one thing, and does provide some protection against manufacturing defects.

ICE DAMS

During the winter, melting snow on our low-pitched roof gets up under the shingles and drips into the soffit under the roof overhang, where the paint is now peeling and the wood is beginning to rot. I think the water must be drawn up under the shingles by capillary action. What can I do to prevent this?

It takes more than capillary action to lift the water high enough to run over the top of the shingles. What happens is this: In freezing weather, sunlight and heat loss from the house melt the snow on the roof, then water runs down and freezes when it reaches the overhang and eavestrough. Eventually the ice builds up and forms a dam that backs the water up under the shingles. If the water backs up far enough it will drip down onto an interior ceiling or run down an inside wall.

A low-pitched roof, a short overhang, and a warm attic are contributing factors. So is the eavestrough itself; in some parts of the country eavestroughs are not used for this reason, but that doesn't always eliminate the problem. Increasing the insulation in the attic will keep the roof colder and reduce the melting. More ventilation in the attic will also help.

During freezing weather, all you can do is chip out openings in the ice dam to let the water run off, but when warm weather returns you have your choice of two relatively permanent remedies. The most common one is to zig-zag an electric heating cable along the lower edge of the roof to keep channels open in the ice dam and the eavestrough. This requires a weatherproof outdoor outlet controlled by an indoor wall switch, preferably one with an indicator light that shows when the heating cable is on, because this uses a fair amount of electricity (about 5 watts per ft).

The other remedy is to have several rows of shingles removed from the bottom of the roof so that a special waterproof, self-sealing, rubberized-asphalt membrane can be applied to the sheathing. When shingles are replaced over this the nail holes in the membrane are sealed automatically. Most roofers are familiar with this method of preventing roof leaks due to ice dams.

LOW-PITCHED ROOF LEAKING

The roof that covers a 14 ft extension at the back of our house has a drop of just 1 ft over this distance. It is covered with two layers of low-slope asphalt shingles, the second applied just a year ago. Each winter the ice and snow buildup on this roof causes water to leak through the den below. The roofer who put it on doesn't know how to correct the problem. Do you have any suggestions?

Your roofer should know that there are no shingles that can be used on a roof with a slope that low (1:14). The minimum roof pitch for low-slope shingles is 1:6. Even roll roofing needs a pitch of at least 1:12. What you require is membrane roofing such as a 4-ply tar-and-gravel roof.

LEAKING ROOF IN A MOBILE HOME

We live in a mobile home with a metal roof that has developed a small hole. How can we patch this?

If the hole is no bigger than $1/4$ in., you can seal it with a dab of fibrated asphalt roofing cement. Up to an inch in diameter you can patch it with a self-stick roof and eavestrough tape that consists of a $1/16$ in. layer of sticky, rubberized asphalt backed with aluminum foil. This is simply cut to size and pressed in place.

Larger holes can be patched with asphalt roofing cement reinforced with aluminum window screen. Spread roofing cement 3 or 4 in. around the hole and cover this with a piece of window screen, then cover the entire patch area with another layer of roofing cement. After this has been allowed to dry for a few days it should be coated with aluminum paint.

METRIC SHINGLES

I plan to put new asphalt shingles on my house this summer, but I'm told that the metric shingles now being used are a different size and can't be applied on top of the old ones. Is this true?

No. There are two ways that metric shingles can be applied over the existing shingles. The simplest is the "nesting" method, which uses the old shingles as a guide for laying the new ones. Cover the exposed bottom row of shingle tabs with a starter strip wide enough to overhang the edge about 1/4 in. The starter strip is made by removing the tabs and about 1 in. from new shingle strips.

The first course of new shingles will butt against the third course of old shingles. Trim the tabs off where they meet the edge of the starter strip. The second course of new shingles butts against the next row of old shingles. Because of the difference in the metric size, the exposed tabs on the bottom row will be about 2 in. shorter than the others, but this won't be noticeable. Continue laying the new shingles butted against the old ones.

The "bridging" method ignores the existing shingle lines and is simply laid like a new roof, following the metric spacing. Because the nesting method makes the exposed shingle tabs a little shorter, it requires 10% to 12% more shingles. On the other hand, the bridging method is more difficult to do and also tends to leave slight ridges every eight courses where the new shingles bridge the old ones.

If this is hard to follow, I suggest you get a copy of the well-illustrated, cartoon-style booklet, *How to Apply Domtar Shingles* (revised metric edition) from your local Domtar distributor. The instructions apply to any metric shingles, of course.

SHADING PLASTIC PATIO ROOF

Some years ago we put a low-pitched roof of corrugated yellow plastic over our patio. This made it a more comfortable place to relax and was a great spot to grow plants. Last year I had to have the roof replaced, and the builder used clear plastic panels instead of yellow ones. When summer came I discovered that the patio was now too hot for us *or* the plants on sunny days. Is there a paint I can use to remedy this?

Greenhouse operators use special white or green shading paints to cut down the sunlight, but these are not very attractive or convenient for residential use. The best remedy is to put roll-up, slatted blinds of bamboo or wood strips on top of the roof. Bamboo blinds are relatively inexpensive and available up to 6 ft in width. They can be opened or closed very easily to suit your needs and the weather. If removed for storage over the winter, a set of bamboo blinds should last for several years. Brushing them with wood preservative at the beginning of the season will prevent a black mildew stain from developing.

SHINGLES DIDN'T SEAL PROPERLY

We wanted to have our roof shingled this summer, but the roofer said it shouldn't be done in hot weather. He did it in late September when the weather was quite cool. During a recent windstorm I noticed that the asphalt shingles were being lifted quite badly.

Contrary to the roofer's advice, asphalt shingles should be applied in weather that is hot enough to soften the adhesive patches used to hold the tabs in place during high winds. These don't stick very well in cool weather, as you can see. The best remedy is to have the roofer come back next summer and press all the shingle tabs down. If the adhesive is not sticky enough at that time, he should put a dab of roofing cement under each tab.

ROOF VALLEY REPAIR

Our country home is L-shaped, and the valley formed where the roofs meet has a metal flashing strip that was damaged during snow removal. Can we replace the valley flashing without removing the shingles?

Because the valley flashing extends under the shingles on both sides, it cannot be replaced without removing the shingles. You should be able to repair the damage, however, if it is not too extensive. Small holes can be covered with dabs of fibrated asphalt roofing compound. Larger holes can be covered with a special patching material that is sold for repairing leaks in eavestroughs. It consists of a sticky asphalt compound about 1/8 in. thick backed with heavy aluminum foil. It comes in rolls of various widths; you just cut off what you need and press it in place. Very large holes can be patched with pieces of galvanized metal embedded in roofing compound.

ROOF VENTS

The asphalt shingles put on our ranch-style house a couple of years ago have started to curl, and some buckling is also evident. The roofer says this is caused by insufficient ventilation in the attic, but we have seven 3x10 roof vents and five 3x12 soffit vents. Isn't this enough? The house has a perimeter floor area of 1800 square feet.

That sounds like a lot, but what matters is not the *number* of vents but their size. The effective area of a screened opening is about half its actual size, so the seven 3x10 roof vents only have a vent area of about 100 square inches, and the five 3x12 soffit vents provide about the same amount. Altogether you have about 1½ square feet of vent area in the attic, which isn't nearly enough. The building code now requires one square foot of attic vent for every 300 square feet of attic floor area, so you will need *six square feet*. You only have a quarter of that.

Instead of putting more vents on your roof, replace two or three of the small ones with 12½ in. square vents and add four 48 in. x 6 in. soffit vents, or their equivalent, to give you an additional four or five square feet of vent area. (Vents are usually stamped with their effective area in square inches.) Alternatively, you could have a ridge vent installed along the peak of your roof.

SIDING

CLEANING ALUMINUM SIDING

The brown aluminum siding on our house has become very dull. Is there any way we can restore the finish to its original bright color and satin sheen?

This is probably due to the normal chalking of exterior paints as they age. To remove this, all you need is a hose, a long-handled scrubbing brush, and a solution of one quart of chlorine laundry bleach, three quarts of water and half a cup of dishwasher detergent. (If you prefer metric, use one litre of bleach, three litres of water and 100ml of detergent.) You will probably need several times this quantity, however.

RESTORING ASBESTOS SIDING

The white asbestos siding on my house has faded to a grey color. How can I restore it?

The siding is probably just dirty. You can clean it with a scrubbing brush and a solution of ¼ cup of trisodium phosphate (TSP) to a gallon of water. Or use a high pressure spray; the equipment is available from most tool rental stores.

If cleaning doesn't make the siding white enough you can apply any exterior latex paint.

NATURAL CEDAR SIDING

We have built a holiday cottage with rough cedar siding that is presently unfinished. We know that this wood weathers to a silvery grey color that many people find attractive, but we would rather keep the cedar in its present reddish brown color. What finish should we apply to do this?

The usual recommendation is to apply a pigmented stain in the shade you want, and this is still good advice. But I have recently learned of a treatment that was developed by the California Redwood Association to retain the natural color of that wood, which is very close to the color of our Western red cedar. The treatment is not a finish, in the usual sense, but a water-repellent preservative that reduces color changes due to weathering, water staining and mildew growth, all of which contribute to the grey color of aged cedar.

The solution consists of 3½ cups of pentachlorophenol wood preservative (5%); 1½ cups of boiled linseed oil; 1 ounce of paraffin wax (melted), and 2 quarts of petroleum solvent or paint thinner. (If you prefer metric, use 800ml of pentachlorophenol wood preservative (5%); 350ml of boiled linseed oil; 30ml of paraffin wax (melted), and 2.6 litres of petroleum solvent or paint thinner.)

Applied generously, one gallon will do about 200 square feet of rough cedar or 400 square feet of smooth cedar. (One litre will do 4 square metres or 8 square metres, respectively.)

If the wood starts to show blotchy discoloration after the first year, scrub it gently with a mild detergent solution, rinse, dry, and then make another generous application of wood preservative solution. The second treatment should last much longer.

MAINTAINING CEDAR SIDING

We have cedar siding on our house and wanted the wood to weather naturally, so

we didn't apply a finish of any kind. Now that the cedar has reached the nice driftwood grey color that we wanted, do we need to apply something to maintain this?

Further aging will not change the color of the wood itself, but in damp or shady areas cedar is sometimes darkened by a mold that looks like soot. This can be prevented by applying a colorless preservative such as pentachlorophenol, which won't affect the color of the wood.

CEMENT SPOTS ON SIDING

Earlier this summer we poured a concrete patio at the back of our house. Unfortunately I neglected to wipe spatters of cement off our white aluminum siding soon enough, and now I can't get them off.

Chip off as much as you can, very carefully, then use a diluted solution of muriatic acid – one part to ten parts water – to dissolve whatever remains. You will have to keep brushing this on until all of the cement is dissolved, and that's a slow job. If it stops foaming, make up a new solution. The factory finish on aluminum siding is unaffected by this solution, but keep it off your skin and protect your eyes with glasses.

DRIVEWAY SEALER ON SIDING

I applied a sealer to my asphalt driveway a few months ago and just as I finished a thunderstorm pelted down and splashed the sealer on the painted siding of my house. Can you tell me how to get this off?

It depends on what kind of sealer you used. If it was an asphalt-based sealer, any petroleum solvent will remove it. Your service station or hardware store has this, and it won't harm the paint

If it was a tar-based sealer, the solvent is toluene, which is the main ingredient in lacquer thinner – and this *may* damage the paint. If it was an acrylic-based driveway sealer you'll have to use a paint remover to get it off, and this *will* damage the paint, of course. Repainting shouldn't be too difficult, however. (See Painting.)

MILDEW ON CEDAR SIDING

The stained cedar siding on my cottage has been discolored by black mildew. How can I remove this and what can I apply to keep if from coming back?

A strong solution of chlorine laundry bleach (Javex, etc.) – about one part to four parts water – will kill the mildew and remove the black stain. If your cottage is located in a shady area close to trees, more mold growth can be expected, but it can be discouraged by applying a colorless wood preservative to the siding. If the siding needs to be re-stained, however, you can use a combination stain/preservative.

NAIL STAINS ON SIDING

Our recently-built house is faced with hardboard siding. The flat-headed nails that the builder used to apply this are now making rust spots on the white paint. He has touched up some of them but the siding still looks pretty bad.

Apparently the builder used the wrong kind of nails. All manufacturers of hardboard siding specify the use of special, *oval-headed, galvanized* siding nails that are designed to prevent this problem.

There is really no way to prevent ungalvanized common nails from rusting through whatever paint is applied. The best remedy is to remove the siding and reapply it correctly. The next best remedy is to use a nailset to drive every flat nailhead into the siding, then cover it with a plastic-based wood filler and repaint. But since the builder did not apply the siding according to the manufacturer's instructions, he should correct it.

STAINING CEDAR SIDING

We are going to put cedar siding on our cottage this summer and would like to stain it. The lumber salesman says we should seal all the knots with shellac first. Is this a good idea?

There is no need to seal the knots in cedar. Unlike most other woods, cedar does not contain pitch pockets that can bleed through paint. Also, shellac would prevent the stain from penetrating the wood the way it's supposed to. Simply apply two coats of the stain directly to the wood.

REPAIRING VINYL SIDING

There is a crack in our vinyl siding. Is there any way I can repair this myself?

The best method is to remove and replace the strip that has been cracked. This can be done quite easily with a "zipper" tool that unlocks the strips, but the work should be undertaken by someone who is familiar with the brand of siding you have.

You can repair the crack reasonably well, however, with one of the vinyl adhesives sold at hardware stores for repairing beach balls, play pools, vinyl eavestroughs and similar products. Use a tooth pick or small brush to apply the adhesive to one edge of the crack, then press the edges together, scrape off the surplus and hold with a strip of masking tape. Remove the tape after a few hours and use very fine sandpaper, if necessary, to remove any adhesive that remains on the surface.

VINYL SIDING HAS BUCKLED

I had vinyl siding put on my house last year, and now I have noticed that several of the siding boards have bowed or buckled in places. Can you tell me what caused this and how to correct it?

It is caused by improper application of the siding. Both metal and vinyl siding expand with heat, and must therefore be nailed *loosely* through the elongated nailing slots that are provided. You should be able to grab one end of a siding strip and move it back and forth half an inch or so as the nails slide in the slots.

Inexperienced or careless workmen often drive the nails in as tightly as if they were putting up lumber. Since this does not allow the vinyl to expand, some sections will bow or buckle when it is heated by the sun. Sometimes this will disappear in cold weather, but more often the distoration becomes set in the vinyl after a period of time, like a wrinkle in a garment, and will not go away by itself. The only remedy is to replace the distored siding. This problem is well known in the siding industry, and your contractor should be prepared to correct his mistake.

WATER STAINS ON CEDAR

The vertical cedar siding on our house is badly watermarked where rain and the garden sprinkler strike it. The stain looks as if the natural pigments in the wood have bled upwards to form a dark brown, jagged line under the window ledges and eaves where the siding is protected from the sun and rain. We would like to remove the watermarks and then obtain an overall silvery grey tone of weathered cedar.

The dark watermarks can be removed with a strong solution of chlorine laundry bleach – one part to three parts water. Then you can apply either a grey pigmented stain or a special

"weathering stain". The latter is a chemical solution, sold by one of the leading stain manufacturers, that speeds up the natural aging process, and does it more evenly than Mother Nature.

SOUNDPROOFING

SOUNDPROOFING BEDROOM

We are having a new house built and would like to soundproof the master bedroom from the rest of the house. The builder has suggested putting fibreglass insulation batts between the studs in the partition walls. Will this do the job?

The addition of fibreglass batts inside a standard frame wall faced on both sides with gypsumboard will reduce sound transmission very little. Good soundproofing can be achieved with fibreglass infill, however, if the gypsumboard is applied on one side of the wall with resilient channels (flexible steel furring strips) to prevent the sound from being transmitted directly through the studs, and gluing a second layer of gypsumboard to at least one side of the wall.

Some sound will still travel through the common floor and ceiling joists, of course, and through the bedroom door, too. You cannot do much about the former, but sealing the door with weatherstripping, particularly at the bottom, will do much to reduce sound leakage there.

SOUNDPROOFING BASEMENT CEILING

I am converting the basement of my old house to a self-contained apartment with a private entrance. I plan to cover the ceiling joists with 4x8 sheets of ½ in. gypsumboard. At present there is only the subfloor and hardwood flooring above – no carpeting – and I would like to know what I can do to soundproof this.

The best way to reduce the impact noises is to put carpeting on the upstairs floor. R12 fibreglass batts pushed up between the joists will reduce sound transmission to some extent, but much of the noise will still be transmitted by the joists. This can be reduced considerably by fastening the gypsumboard to the joists with something called "resilient channel", a springlike metal strip that isolates the panels from the floor structure.

Weight is also a factor in lowering sound transmision, so ⅝ in. (16mm) gypsumboard panels would be better than ½ in. (13mm). And the soundproofing will be even better if you apply two layers of gypsumboard, the second at right angles to the first and attached with panel adhesive instead of screws.

SOUNDPROOFING FAMILY ROOM

We are building an addition on our house that will include a family room with an adjoining bedroom. Since we have a large family and teenage children we are very concerned about sound transmission between these rooms. Our builder suggests using a staggered stud wall with fibreglass batts woven horizontally between the studs and gypsumboard panelling on both sides. You once recommended fastening the gypsumboard to the studs with resilient metal channel; would that improve the soundproofing of this wall?

That works well on a standard stud wall but provides little benefit on a staggered stud wall like this, since there is no direct contact between the two wall surfaces, anyway. A substantial improvement in soundproofing can be achieved, however, by adding a second layer of gypsumboard to both sides of this wall. It will also help if you bed the 2x6 bottom plate on two beads of resilient caulking compound, and also use this in the small gap that should be left between the gypsumboard and the floor, ceiling and adjoining walls. When you are striving for a high level of soundproofing like this, even tiny cracks can spoil a good job. Although this wall will be an excellent sound barrier, you will still have the problem of sound transmission through the common floor and ceiling joists. Isolating these is a difficult problem.

SILENCING A HEAT PUMP

When our neighbor had a swimming pool installed in his back yard last summer he moved his heat pump to the side of the house, about 10 ft from ours and right below the master bedroom windows on the second floor. We had never noticed any noise from the heat pump before, but now it sounds like a car engine running outside the bedroom all night. Is there some kind of a fence I can build to reduce this noise?

Sound travels in a straight line, so the fence would have to be high enough to hide the heat pump from view from your bedroom windows. It would also have to be made of a heavy, sound-absorbing material such as concrete

blocks. Building regulations would not permit a property-line wall this high, I'm sure, but it could be much lower if your neighbor built it on his side, close to the noisy fan and compressor unit. Your neighbor may also be able to get a special sound baffle added to the heat pump to reduce the noise level.

About all you can do on your side to reduce the noise is add another pane to the inside or outside of your bedroom windows. This could cut the sound level about in half, however. Heavy drapes would also help. But if none of the above steps corrects the problem, you may be able to get a court order requiring your neighbor to move the heat pump to the back of his property again.

NOISY NEIGHBOR

Our neighbor's driveway is right under our bedroom window, and since he is on shift work he often comes and goes when we are, or would like to be, sleeping. It is particularly annoying in winter when he shovels snow off the driveway to get his car in or out. Our wood frame house was built in the '60s, so I don't think we have much insulation in the walls. I was thinking of removing the siding and sheathing and putting batt insulation between the studs. Will this be enough to keep out the noise from our neighbor's driveway, or do I have to add another frame wall?

The windows are more of a problem than the walls. Even in the '60s, some insulation was required in frame walls, and you will probably find that you have 2½ in. batts there – adding more will not make much difference in their sound transmission rating. And since the windows already let in more sound than the walls do, they determine the noise level in your bedroom. There is no point in having the walls more soundproof than the windows, in other words.

The best you can do with the windows is to seal them completely (no air leakage at all), add a sealed storm pane either outside or inside (or both, if you have no storm pane now) and hang heavy drapes over them. This combination will give the windows a sound transmission rating just about equal to a 2x4 frame wall with some batt insulation. This still leaves the problem of ventiltion in the bedroom, of course. If you open a window even a crack, the noise will come in about as loud as ever. As you can see, the problem is a lot more difficult than it sounds. It would be a lot easier to move your bedroom.

SOUNDPROOFING A PARTY WALL

We own a semi-detached home and have just acquired new neighbors who entertain a lot and like loud music. There is just a frame wall between us, and the noise is driving me crazy. (Now I know why they call it a "party wall".) Is there anything we can do on our side of the wall to lower the noise level?

A considerable reduction in the noise level can be achieved. Apply 2x2 furring strips horizontally to the top and bottom of the wall and about every 24 in. in between. Next, place a sound-absorbing material such as 2½ in. or 2¾ in. fibreglass batts between the furring strips, holding them to the wall with construction adhesive, if necessary. Attach ⅝ in. (16mm) gypsumboard panelling to the furring strips with a spring-like metal fastening strip called "resilient channel". A second layer of gypsumboard should then be applied with mastic adhesive.

A gap of ⅛ in. should be left between the edges of the gypsumboard and the adjoining floor, ceiling and walls to prevent the direct transmission of sound vibrations to the new wall. Fill the gap with an acoustic caulking compound.

The combination of a 2 in. air space, the sound-absorbing fibreglass, and a 1¼ in. layer of heavy gypsumboard panelling suspended on resilient supports makes this about as soundproof a wall as can be achieved, but some sounds will still be transmitted through the common framework of the two units, particularly the floor and ceiling joists. There is no practical way to eliminate this.

TRAFFIC NOISE

I live in a bungalow and the large windows in my bedroom face a street that has become very noisy in recent years. The windows have sealed double-glazing and I keep them closed, but a lot of noise still gets through. What can I do to reduce it?

An extra storm pane on the inside or outside will help. (The larger the air space the better the sound reduction.) You can also obtain roll-up exterior blinds or shutters that are controlled from the inside and are designed to provide soundproofing as well as insulation and security. Heavy drapes inside will also help, of course.

There are some landscaping tricks that will reduce traffic noise, too. Evergreen trees will block a lot of sound. Building an earth berm between the windows and the street, and topping this with evergreen shrubs, will also be effec-

tive. Even a hedge will help, although it may take a few years to become effective. A faster remedy is to build a sound barrier wall of concrete block between the house and the traffic, but local building regulations may not permit this.

STAIN REMOVAL

ALUMINUM POT BLACKENED

Can you tell me how to clean an aluminum saucepan that has turned black on the inside because of something that was boiled in it?

A steel wool soap pad will remove the tarnish, but an easier way to do it is to fill the saucepan with water above the tarnish line, bring it to a boil and add a heaping teaspoon of cream of tartar, which you probably have among your baking supplies. Continue simmering and the aluminum will become cleaner than you have ever seen it.

DISCOLORED BATHTUB

After removing some plastic decals that had been on the bottom of our bathtub for many years we discovered that the porcelain enamel under the decals was still snow white, but the rest of the tub had turned slightly grey. None of the cleaners I have used, including a strong solution chlorine laundry bleach, have done any good.

Try a paste made of cream of tartar and hydrogen peroxide, applied with a stiff brush.

BLACK STAIN ON DISH MAT

A large, black stain has appeared on a light-colored rubber drain mat I use under the dish rack beside the sink. Scrubbing with soap and water won't take it off. What should I use?

A strong solution of chlorine laundry bleach – about one ounce to four ounces of water – will remove the black stain, which is actually a mold growth. To keep it from forming, wipe the drain mat occasionally with the bleach solution.

BLACK WATER STAINS ON WOOD

Wet boots were left on the oak floor in our hallway, and this has left black marks in the wood that will not come off with anything I have tried. Do you have a magic remedy for removing this ugly black stain?

It is one of the few problems I DO have a magic remedy for. A concentrated solution of oxalic acid will bleach out this stain. Oxalic acid crystals are available from any drug store; they may even have it on the shelves labelled as Rust Remover, which it also is. (The label will say: "Contains oxalic acid".) Or you may find it among the cleaning materials at your supermarket under the name of ZUD Rust Remover.

Dissolve a teaspoon in half a cup of water to make a concentrated solution (don't worry if it doesn't all dissolve). Soak a piece of cloth in this solution and place it over the stain. Check every five minutes or so and remove as soon as the black stain has disappeared. Wipe with a damp cloth or sponge and dry with a paper towel.

BLOOD STAINS

I have a lovely old quilt that has been washed a number of times but still has some small blood stains on it. Do you know of any way I can remove these?

Cold water will remove fresh blood stains very quickly, but they are difficult to get out once they have dried. An old remedy that often works is to apply hydrogen peroxide to the stains. This foams up and loosens the dried blood so it can be removed by washing. A reader also told me that meat tenderizer will remove blood stains, which sounds logical. Ammonia has also been recommended. Enzyme laundry detergents were very effective on blood stains, but I don't think these are available any longer.

CONCRETE STAINS ON CAR TOP

There is a leak in the concrete ceiling of the underground garage of our apartment building, right over the spot where I had to park my car recently. This has left white spots on the top of the car, and none of the cleaners I have tried will remove them. Whatever the material is, it forms little icicle-like drops on the ceiling. These break off easily and I have enclosed one for your inspection. Other residents in the building have the same problem and we would certainly be glad to learn how to remove these stains without harming the car finish.

A test of the sample you send confirms what I suspected: it is a lime deposit that dissolves readily (but slowly) in vinegar, which won't harm auto body paint. I suggest you fold a paper towel into a small pad, soak it with vinegar and place it on the stain for as long as it takes to dissolve the lime deposit.

EGG STAINS ON STUCCO

Some months ago vandals threw eggs on our stucco house and we are having great difficulty getting the stains off. Can you tell us what to use?

Liquid drain cleaner or a strong solution of lye should do it. I would dilute the liquid drain cleaner with an equal quantity of water first, but if this is not strong enough, use it full strength. If you want to make your own solution, dissolve one 9½-ounce (280 grams) can of lye in two quarts or two litres of water.

These are all strong caustic solutions and should be handled with great care. Wear rubber gloves and glasses and be careful to keep the solution off everything but the stucco. Keep a wet rag handy to wipe any splatters off your skin.

The caustic solutions will also remove any paint that is on the stucco, but it will probably be necessary to repaint it after it has been cleaned, in any case. Any exterior latex paint can be used.

FELT PEN INK ON VINYL

How can I remove a black felt pen mark from white vinyl upholstery?

Special removers are available at some stationery stores, but you can do the job about as well with rubbing alcohol, wood alcohol (methyl hydrate), vodka, or even hair spray.

STAINS ON FIBREGLASS BATHTUB

I am having trouble removing stains from my fibreglass bathtub. What is the proper treatment to remove these?

The smooth, colored surface of fibreglass fixtures like this consists of a tough polyester-styrene "gel coat" that must meet CSA standards for resistance to stain or damage from common household chemicals. Whatever stains you have are probably just on the surface, and you should be able to remove them with a gentle abrasive such as automobile rubbing compound or even brass polish.

GREEN STAIN IN SINK

A green stain has formed on the bottom of our white sink. What causes this and how can I remove it?

The first thing you should do is put new washers in the taps to stop them dripping, which is the immediate cause of the discoloration. The green stain, however, comes from copper salts dissolved in the water, usually because it is too acidic (a problem that is related to acid rain).

Municipal water supplies are not usually treated for acidity because it is not harmful to humans (soft drinks and fruit juices are much more acidic) but it can be strong enough to corrode copper pipes. To correct it you can install a device that feeds a harmless neutralizing chemical into your water supply. These are available from companies that sell water softening equipment. They will also test your water without charge, or you can do it yourself wth a garden or swimming pool pH testing kit. If the pH reading is below 6.5 you should consider intalling a neutralizing unit.

But another possible cause for the dissolved copper salts is corrosion due to the small electric current that is produced when two dissimilar metals such as copper and iron are joined in the plumbing system. Such connections should only be made with special "dielectric" fittings. A plumber can install these now if this is your problem.

The stain itself, often called "green rust", can be removed quite easily with lemon juice and salt. Just squeeze lemon juice on the stain and then sprinkle with salt. Some household copper cleaners will also remove the green copper stains.

LEAF STAINS ON PATIO

Leaves that fell on my new concrete patio last fall have left dark brown stains that won't wash off. How can I remove them?

They will fade away by themselves in a few months, but you can hasten the process by applying a fairly strong solution of chlorine laundry bleach - say one part to three parts water.

OIL STAIN ON PATIO

I spilled some cooking oil on my concrete patio, and my efforts to remove it only spread it around, I'm afraid. What should I use to get rid of it?

Buy about half a pound (225 grams) of powdered white chalk from a hardware store. Mix this with enough petroleum solvent (Varsol, Shell Sol, etc.) to make a paste. Spread this on the oil stain about a quarter of an inch thick and cover it with polyethylene film or plastic food wrap held down around the edges with masking tape. Leave for a couple of hours, then remove the plastic and let the paste dry thoroughly to draw the dissolved oil up into the chalk. When you brush this off, most of the oil will go with it. Repeat as necessary.

PROTECTING MARBLE

We have a table with a pale blue marble top that is picking up stains. Is there anything we can apply to the marble to prevent this?

An application of white paste wax or one of the clear acrylic floor polishes will protect marble from water-based stains.

VINYL STAINED BY RUBBER MAT

We have been using a rubber-backed mat on the white vinyl floor in front of the kitchen sink. Now we have discovered that this has made a yellowish stain on the vinyl, and nothing we have tried will remove it. Any suggestions?

Such stains sometimes can be taken off with nail polish remover, I am told. A strong solution of chlorine laundry bleach, say one part to two parts water, is another possibility. Apply with a pad of #0000 steel wool.

RUST STAIN IN TOILET BOWL

An iron fitting in my toilet tank caused the bowl to become badly stained with rust. I replaced the fitting with a plastic one, but no matter what I try I can't get the rust stain out of the porcelain bowl. Do you have a remedy for this?

Oxalic acid is the best remedy for rust stains, and I have recently learned of a good way to use it for this problem. Remove about half of the water from the toilet bowl, then fill it with hot water and a rounded tablespoon of oxalic acid crystals (available from any drugstore). The hot water speeds the action, and the rust stain will disappear almost immediately.

NAIL STAINS ON FENCE

Our property is bordered on one side by a wooden fence put up by the developer. Apparently he didn't use galvanized nails, and now there are rust streaks running down the boards. We want to re-stain the fence, but would like to know how to prevent the rust stains from reappearing.

The best remedy is to remove the fence boards, use sandpaper to take off the rust stains, then reassemble the fence with hot-dipped galvanized nails. If that's too much of a job, simply hammer each nail firmly into the board and then cover the head with a dab of alkyd paint in a color close to the stain you are going to use.

RUST STAIN ON UPHOLSTERY

I cleaned my beige velvet chesterfield with a foam shampoo, and when it dried I discovered there were rust stains around the buttons. Can you tell me how I can remove these?

Get a small quantity of citric acid from your drug store - or "sour salt" from your grocer; it's the same thing. Dissolve a heaping teaspoon of this in about two ounces of water to make a concentrated solution. Apply this to the rust stain with a brush or sponge, sprinkle it with table salt, then hold a steam iron just above the fabric to steam the spot. The combination of citric acid, salt and heat will quickly bleach out the rust stain.

Check the process on a hidden part of the upholstery first to make sure it won't bleach the fabric too. Any citric acid you have left over can be used to make lemonade.

SALT STAINS

How can I remove salt stains from the rug in my front hall?

Sponge them with vinegar, then rinse and dry.

REMOVING TAR STAINS

We were having a new tar-and-gravel roof put on our garage, and somehow I managed to get a little on one of my suits. Nothing I've tried seems to remove this. Can you tell me how to get it off?

A built-up roof like this can be made of either tar or asphalt. They look much the same but require different solvents. Asphalt can be removed with a petroleum solvent such as Varsol or one of the non-flammable chlorinated dry-cleaning solvents like per-, tri-, or tetra- chloroethylene, available at any drug store.

If neither of these works, the spot on your suit must be tar. The solvent for this is toluene, which is the main constituent of lacquer thinner, available at any hardware or paint store. This is *very* inflammable, so use it only in a well ventilated room - or better still, outdoors.

VENTILATION

VENTILATING THE ATTIC

In a recent column you mentioned the importance of adequate ventilation in the attic to prevent condensation and frost under the roof. I am planning to add more insulation up there and I would like to know what I should do, or not do, to assure proper ventilation first.

For many years now, the building code has required a minimum of one square foot of open vent in the attic for every 300 square feet of floor area, but most older homes have a lot less. Ideally, half of this should be along the lower edge of the roof, such as under the eaves or soffit, and the other half high up on the roof. A ridge vent that fits over the peak of the roof is probably the best type to use here, but triangular gable vents or the common mushroom roof vents will also do the job. (Power-driven roof vents are only necessary in rare cases where the job cannot be done with conventional vents, otherwise the cost of buying and installing them is not justified.)

All vents should be stamped with their effective area, which is usually a lot less than you expect. The common 7½ in. diameter roof vent, for instance, has an effective area of only 37 square inches - it takes four of them to provide one square foot of vent area. You would need eight of them, plus an equivalent area of soffit vents, to ventilate a 1200-square-foot attic. Individual roof vents with an effective area of one square foot are available.

You must be sure, too, that the insulation you put in the attic doesn't block the air flow from the soffit vents. This can be done by inserting inexpensive cardboard or plastic chutes between the insulation and the roof. Ask about these where you buy your insulation.

BATHROOM VENTED TO ATTIC

We just bought a 5-year-old house and have discovered that the ceiling fan in the upstairs bathroom vents directly into the attic. Is this a good idea? If not, should I vent it through the roof or an outside wall?

This can cause serious condensation problems in the attic. For many years it has been against the buildng code to vent an exhaust fan into the attic. Putting it up through the roof isn't a good idea, either, because moisture will condense inside the cold duct and run back into the bathroom fan. Wrapping the duct with insulation won't stop this entirely.

It's much better to run the exhaust duct horizontally between the joists to a vent under the roof overhang. Remove the insulation between the joists and put it on top of the duct.

DUCTLESS RANGE HOOD

During the winter my kitchen windows steam up whenever I cook. I can't find any place to put the ductwork for a range hood exhaust fan, so ! was thinking of installing a ductless range hood. Will this reduce the humidity?

No. It simply recirculates the air through filters that remove some of the oils, fats and cooking odors, but it does nothing to get rid of the humidity. Only ventilation will do that. An exhaust fan installed in an outside wall of the kitchen, without any ductwork, will do the job very well, however. It should have a capacity of 2 CFM (cubic feet per minute) for each square foot of kitchen floor area.

EXHAUST FAN NOT WORKING

The exhaust fan in our bathroom ceiling doesn't seem to work properly anymore. The walls drip when someone has a shower and the fan doesn't appear to be drawing out any air at all. It runs at a good speed, however, and doesn't appear to be dirty. What can be the problem?

Something must be blocking the air flow. It could be a stuck flap valve on the outlet of the fan housing. (You may have to remove the fan to check this.) If not, check the ductwork in the attic, taking it apart if necessary. If the vent goes out a side wall, look for a bird's nest inside the duct – this is a common problem. Check the flap valve on the outside of the exhaust vent to make sure it isn't stuck. The trouble has to be somewhere along the ductwork.

DRAFT FROM EXHAUST FAN

The range hood in our kitchen contains an exhaust fan that is vented through an outside wall. On windy days we have trouble with cold air coming in through the range hood.

The outside vent cap should contain a weighted flap or damper that will stay closed when the fan is not running. This can't be working properly. Three things could be wrong. The damper may be stuck; try loosening it with a little penetrating oil applied to the hinge pins. The damper may be bent; see if you can straighten it. Or there may not be enough weight on the damper to keep it closed when the wind is blowing; use rubber cement to attach one or more metal washers to the damper.

If these steps don't correct the problem you may have to buy a new outside vent cap. Get one with a locking device that holds the damper shut until an inner shutter is opened by fan pressure. This kind is much more airtight.

VENTILATING A MOBILE HOME

During cold weather a lot of water drips down through the ceiling exhaust fan in the kitchen of our mobile home. What causes this and how can we stop it?

Warm, humid household air is condensing on the cold walls of the exhaust fan duct and running back into the kitchen. This will happen even when the fan is not running, because the lightweight damper that is supposed to keep the vent closed when the fan is not running cannot resist the combined upward pressure of warm air and wind suction. This also results in a significant heat loss.

A much better location for an exhaust fan in a mobile home is high on a wall, with a 3 in. diameter metal duct extending down the wall, through the floor (where it should be tightly caulked) and out through the skirting around the crawlspace. The present ceiling fan can be disconnected and moved to this position, and the ceiling hole stuffed with fibreglass insulation and covered with polyethylene vapor barrier.

TWO VENT FANS – ONE DUCT

We have two bathrooms back to back, and only one of them has an exhaust fan in the ceiling. Would it be possible to connect an exhaust fan in the second bathroom to the same duct?

An exhaust fan in an outside wall works much better, and that would be the best location for a fan in the second bathroom, if this can be done. If not, you should be able to connect a second ceiling fan to the existing duct. The 4 in. duct that is usually installed is large enough to handle the air flow from two bathroom ceiling fans. I would suggest, however, that you check the anti-backflow damper in each exhaust fan unit to make sure it is sealed tightly when it is closed, otherwise air could be blown from one bathroom to the other when the fan is used. You may have to remove the fan to get at the damper, but that's not difficult.

WALLPAPER

PAPERING WITH GRASSCLOTH

I want to paper my hallway with grasscloth but have been told that this is very tricky to work with. I have done some wallpapering, but would like to know what special precautions I must take with grasscloth.

Grasscloth is easier to work with than most wallpapers. There is no pattern to worry about, for one thing, and little wastage, because lengths can be joined invisibly at any point. The only special instructions are to use a clear, non-staining adhesive and to hang every other strip upside down to avoid a shading pattern caused by the way grasscloth is dyed during manufacture. (You will notice a dark dye stain running down one side of the paper backing; use this as a guide when you are reversing alternate strips.) I found it easier to apply the paste to the wall instead of the back of the paper, but it can be done either way. Do just enough for one strip at a time to keep the adhesive from drying out too fast. Although grasscloth is quite stiff, it can be bent around outside and inside corners easily enough. A short length of board helps to fold it sharply around an outside corner or push it into an inside corner.

LOOSE WALLPAPER

The window wall in our bedroom has been papered for a few years, and I recently noticed that the paper is coming loose along the top of the wall. What can I use to glue this back so it will come off when I want to replace the paper?

Use one of the glue sticks that are sold at stationery stores. These have a waxy consistency that holds paper very well but doesn't harden the way most liquid adhesives do. Besides, they are very easy to use. Just peel back the loose paper and rub the stick either on the wall or the back of the paper, then press it in place.

The problem is probably caused by condensation forming along the top of the wall during cold weather, and this is due to too much humidity in the house. More ventilation is the remedy.

PAPERING OVER HARDBOARD

Our basement rec room is panelled with one of the simulated woodgrain hardboards. I applied prepasted wallpaper to this some months ago, and now it has pulled away in several places. What did I do wrong?

This type of panelling has a very smooth surface that wallpaper adhesive doesn't stick to very well. It should be given a coat of alkyd or other oil-based primer before the paper is applied.

PAPERING OVER PLYWOOD

The kitchen in our cottage is panelled with plywood, to which a mixture of boiled linseed oil and turpentine was applied many years ago. I would like to paper these walls now. How should I prepare the plywood surface for papering?

Fill any open joints or other holes with one of the premixed plaster patching materials, then sand these smooth before papering. The oiled plywood itself needs no further preparation. I suggest you use a washable vinyl-coated paper, applying it with the adhesive recommended by the manufacturer.

REMOVING WALLPAPER

How can I remove wallpaper from drywall panelling without damaging the paper face of the gypsumboard? We are tired of the pattern and want to paint the wall instead.

Most wallpaper sold in recent years has been dry strippable. You only need to lift up a corner and then peel it off. If you don't have this kind of wallpaper, and it is stuck firmly to the wall, it's better just to leave it there and paint over it. If there are any open seams fill them first with a plaster patching compound and a 2 in. putty knife.

PAPERING V-JOINT PANELLING

I would like to paper a wall that is covered with V-joint wood panelling that has a very dark stain and a shiny finish. How can I fill the joints between the boards to get a smooth surface for the wallpaper?

You don't have to fill the V-joints but there are two other things you must do. First roughen the finish with sandpaper to remove the gloss and provide a better grip for the adhesive. Then apply a heavy grade of "lining paper", a plain, plasticized paper that is strong enough to bridge cracks, grooves and other holes, and provides a smooth base for the decorative paper. Lining paper is applied with wallpaper paste but doesn't have to be trimmed and can be laid either vertically or horizonatatly. It is available at any wallpaper store, but be sure to get the heavy grade.

WALLPAPER PEELING

I applied a prepasted paper over the painted walls in my living room. A strip of paper above the baseboard heater and below the window peeled off shortly afterwards, and so has a second strip I applied. What am I doing wrong and how can I correct it?

The peelable adhesive used on prepasted wallpaper is not very strong, and does not take much to weaken it enough to cause a problem like this. Perhaps there is a slight film of dirt above the baseboard heater. Or the wall may have been finished with a latex paint that was not sealed before the paper was applied. Add to this the faster drying of the adhesive on the warm wall over the heater and you have a likely explanation for your problem. But whatever the cause, the simple remedy is to reglue the peeled paper to the wall with regular wallpaper adhesive.

REMOVING VINYL WALLPAPER

We peeled the vinyl-coated paper off our bathroom walls, and it has left a surface like fuzzy blotting paper. How do we prepare this for the new wallcovering we want to put up?

Only the printed surface layer of vinyl-coated paper comes off when you peel it. The backing paper stays on the wall, and that is what you have now. This can be papered over if you use wallpaper paste, but if you want to use pre-pasted paper, or paint the wall, it is better to remove the backing paper. You can do this by wetting it with wallpaper remover then scraping the softened paper off the wall with a broad putty knife. If the wall was properly primed, the backing paper will come off easily and the new paper can be applied directly. If you don't a see white prime coat on the wall, however, apply an oil-based (alkyd) primer before you put up the new wallcovering.

WINDOWS

WINDOW CLEANER

We have a lot of windows in our house, including one complete window wall, and I am finding it very expensive buying the commercial spray-bottle cleaners, although they work very well. Can you give me the formula for a solution I could make up myself?

A couple of years ago one of the U.S. consumer magazines found the following solution at least as good as any of the commercial products they tested: 5 ounces of sudsy ammonia, 20 ounces of isopropyl rubbing alcohol, a teaspoon of liquid dish detergent and 3½ quarts of water. (If you prefer metric, it's 110ml of sudsy ammonia, 450ml of isopropyl alcohol, 5ml of detergent, and 3 litres of water.) The cost works out to about 70 cents a quart or 80 cents a litre.

LEAKING WINDOW

During a recent severe wind and rain storm a lot of water seeped in around our kitchen window. This happened a couple of other times and we blamed it on an overflowing eavestrough, but we have kept this clear ever since.

This is probably caused by water getting in around the outside of the window frame, and the remedy is to apply caulking there. But it could also be caused by rain driving up under the shingles and leaking down inside the wall. The remedy for this is to put a dab of asphalt roofing cement or hot-melt glue under each of the shingle tabs along the bottom 3 ft or so of the roof.

REMOVING REFLECTIVE FILM FROM WINDOWS

We applied reflective film to our bedroom windows a few years ago in an effort to reduce the heat build up there during the summer. It did some good, but we found that it also keeps the winter sun from warming this room. Now we would like to remove the reflective film from the glass and use venetian blinds or shades instead. How can we do this?

That depends on what type of film you have. The newest type has a release adhesive that peels off the glass cleanly and easily. An earlier type had a gummy adhesive, some of which remains on the glass after the film has been peeled off. This can be removed with water and a nylon scouring pad. The oldest type must be soaked with water before it can be peeled off the glass. The best way to do this is to apply sheets of wet newspaper or cloth to the window for about an hour, keeping them wet with a spray bottle, if necessary. When the adhesive has softened, the film should peel off the glass in one sheet. Use a wet sponge to remove any adhesive left on the glass.

REPAIRING WINDOW BLINDS

We put new window shades in our bedroom about a year ago, and twice we have had to put new pins in the ends of the rollers. The pins have worn through, and new ones are very hard to find. What could be causing this?

I suspect that the pins are turning in cheap metal brackets with sharp edges. Replace the brackets with ones that contain a nylon bushing. They only cost a few cents more than the plain metal ones.

If you can't find new pins, make your own by driving a 2½ in. common nail a little more than 1 in. into the hole in the end of the roller, then cut it off with a hacksaw, leaving about ⅜ in. protruding. Before you put the shade back in the brackets, loosen the tension of the roller spring by unwinding the shade about half way down the window.

ALUMINUM WINDOWS

The windows on the south side of my 34-year-old house have wood frames that are beginning to rot. I am thinking of replacing them with double-glazed aluminum windows like I have at the back of my house, but these produce puddles of water on the sill all winter because of condensation on the metal frames. How can I prevent this?

Metal conducts heat much faster than wood, so is a lot colder in winter. The way to overcome this is to get aluminum windows that have a layer of insulation, called a "thermal break", between the inside and outside sections of the metal frame. This will keep the inside surface of the aluminum from getting cold enough to cause condensation to form - although this could still happen if you let the humidity in your house get too high during very cold weather.

FREEING STUCK WINDOW

After recent rains, one of my double-hung windows seems to have swollen shut and I am unable to open it.

A couple of weeks of dry weather should loosen it. If not, you can free the window by removing one of the strips of stop molding that is holding the sash in place on the room side. It may be necessary to have someone push the sash from the outside, however, to remove it.

If the side rails of the sash have swelled, move the stop molding back about ¹/₁₆ in. when you replace it. If the window is too wide, sand or plane the sides for a better fit. Rubbing a block of paraffin wax in the side channels will lubricate them and help to keep the window sash running smoothly.

MOISTURE INSIDE THERMAL WINDOWS

Our house is eight years old and we are beginning to get moisture or condensation between the panes of our sealed, double-glazed thermal windows. We have been told that we can eliminate this by adding storm windows on the outside. Is this true?

Partly. Adding a storm window will make the outside pane of the sealed thermal unit a little warmer, and this will sometimes be enough to prevent condensation inside the double glazing. But moisture will still appear when the outside temperature gets low enough.

The problem is caused by failure of the air seal around the thermal unit, allowing humid air and dirt to get inside it. There is no practical way to correct this; sooner or later the thermal windows will have to be replaced.

TRIPLE vs DOUBLE THERMAL WINDOWS

The salesman for a prefabricated home company told me that all the windows in their houses were triple-glazed except for those facing south. He claimed that the third pane would keep out solar heat. When I talked to some window manufacturers about this, they said it would be better to have triple windows on all sides. Now I'm confused.

The home salesman has the right idea but the wrong explanation. A triple-glazed window provides more insulation than a double-glazed window wherever it's located, and only keeps out a little bit more solar heat. As far as heat conservation is concerned, you would be better off with triple windows throughout. But most heat is lost through windows on the north side, and a triple window will pay for itself much faster here. On the south side of the house even a double-glazed window provides a net heat *gain* over the winter, and I don't think the extra cost of triple-glazing here is justified.

DRAINING A WINDOW WELL

During a recent rainstorm the window wells around our basement filled with water, some of which came inside. Is there some way we can put drains in the window wells?

The job is simple enough, but a lot of work. It's just a matter of running a drainage line down to the perimeter tile system that you should have around the bottom of the foundation wall. You'll have to remove the corrugated metal or other cribbing that holds the earth away from the window well, then dig down to the foundation footings and the drainage tile. Insert a tee connection here so a vertical tile line can be run up to the window well. Put these drainage tiles in place as you refill the excavation and tamp the earth around them. When you reach the bottom of the window well, replace the cribbing and cover the open tile with ½ in. wire screen or "hardware cloth", then add a couple of inches of gravel.

An easier solution, however, is to put a moulded, transparent plastic cover over the window well. These are available at most building supply stores.

WOOD

ALGAE ON CEDAR DECK

I'm having a problem with green algae growing on the shady areas of a cedar deck at the back of my house. Will this harm the wood? If so, how can I get rid of the algae and what should I do to keep it from coming back?

Because the algae holds a lot of moisture, it promotes wood decay and should be removed. It is also very slippery. Scrape off as much as you can, then scrub the deck with a stiff brush and a solution of one part chlorine laundry bleach to three parts water, plus one tablespoon of *dishwasher* detergent per quart of solution. When the deck is clean and dry, apply a clear wood preservative.

BEAMS ROTTING

We have an old house and recently discovered that one of the beams in the basement was so badly decayed that it had to be replaced. Now I have noticed that adjacent timbers are also showing signs of decay. How can we stop this?

Wood must be damp for the decay fungus to grow. Even the so-called "dry rot" fungus will not grow in wood that contains less than 22% moisture by weight. The first step is to find and eliminate the source of the moisture, which may be a plumbing leak, poor drainage around the foundation walls, an unvented clothes dryer, or an uncovered earth floor.

A generous application of wood preservative will prevent decay organisms from becoming established on the surface of wood that is presently uninfected, such as the new beam, but it will not prevent the decay spreading in wood where it is already growing. The only way to do that is to keep the wood dry, or replace it with good wood.

CEDAR TURNING BLACK

Our cedar log cottage is gradually turning black. How can we get rid of this and keep it from coming back? We like the natural color of the logs.

The black stain is caused by a mold growth that probably comes from nearby trees – which may also provide the shade that encourages it. It can be removed with a strong solution of chlorine laundry bleach, one part to four parts water. When this dries, apply a wood preservative to discourage further mold growth.

HOW BIG IS A CORD?

In discussing the comparative costs of different fuels, you recently referred to a "full cord" of wood. Can you tell me the exact size of this?

A cord of wood is a stack measuring 4 ft x 4 ft x 8 ft. The wood usually comes in lengths from 16 in. to 24 in., but sometimes it's cut as short as 12 in. The term "face cord", although not officially recognized, is sometimes used to mean a 4 ft x 8 ft stack of firewood cut to one of these lengths, which means that it will actually be anywhere from one-quarter to one-half of a real cord. It's very important to know the size of the wood, in other words, when buying a face cord. Even then, the only way to be sure of what you're getting is to stack the wood up and measure it as soon as you get it.

WOOD DECK ROTTING

We have a wood deck extending outside our house from the living room. Some of the floor boards are rotting. They are spaced about a quarter of an inch apart, and examination has shown that there is a small amount of decay on top of some of the beams that support the decking, too. I would like to know if I should replace the floor boards with plywood and then apply some kind of waterproofing material over it. And what can I use to stop the decay in the beams?

The spaced decking you have will last longer than plywood. One reason is that any waterproofing membrane you can apply is likely to crack or be punctured by chair legs, etc., in a location like this. Then water will get underneath and you will *really* have a decay problem.

Replace the rotten floor boards or planks with pressure-treated "outdoor" lumber. As the decking is removed, brush the beams with pentachlorophenol or other colorless wood preservative. Apply this two or three times, letting it sink in well each time. Then apply the new decking, which should be left unfinished.

MATCHING FENCE BOARDS

The rough cedar boards on our fence have weathered to an attractive driftwood grey. A few of the boards were broken recently and I have to replace them. How can I get the new lumber to match the weathered fence?

Leading stain manufacturers put out a wide range of colors, including some that duplicate the tone of weathered cedar. You can mix your own stain quite easily, however, with equal parts of boiled linseed oil and petroleum solvent plus black pigment. A tube of lampblack, available in the paint section of most hardware stores, will be enough to color several litres of stain. But add the pigment slowly, mix thoroughly, and test the stain on scraps of cedar as you prepare it.

"WOOD FLOUR"

A folder put out by one of the white resin glue manufacturers says you can make your own plastic wood or filler by mixing this adhesive with "wood flour". None of the hardware stores I've been to carries this. Where can I get it?

Wood flour is just sanding dust. You make it yourself by sanding the wood you want to fill. Just mix this with the adhesive to make a matching filler.

WOOD FOUNDATIONS

We are planning to build a new home and our builder has suggested using a foundation made of preserved wood. He tells us this has several advantages over concrete, but we have never heard of it and are concerned about its durability. Can you give us your opinion of wood foundations, and any other information that would help us make up our minds?

You have probably seen a number of houses with wood foundations without being aware of it. Many thousands have been built in Canada and the United States since the first research model was constructed in an Ottawa subdivision in 1961. This and other early models have been monitored carefully ever since and are still in excellent condition.

Preserved wood foundations have been approved by Canada Mortgage and Housing Corporation and most provincial building codes for many years. Strict standards for their construction have been in force since 1976. Wood foundations are built very much like wood frame walls but are thicker and stronger. All the framing and sheathing lumber is pressure-impregnated with wood preservatives to higher standards than required for other uses. The foundation walls rest on treated wood footings supported on a gravel drainage bed that seems to work much better than the conventional perimeter drain tile system. The basement floor can be concrete or wood. Because frame foundation walls can be insulated even better than the walls in the main living areas, the basement space is at least as warm, dry and comfortable as the rest of the house, and heating costs are lower than they would be with a conventional poured concrete or block foundation.

Comparative construction costs vary with different areas and builders, so you will have to obtain this information yourself. One of the main benefits for builders is the fact that wood foundations can be constructed by their regular framing crew. They can also be put up even in the coldest weather, so winter building can proceed without delay.

More detailed information is contained in a 40-page booklet, *Preserved Wood Foundations* (WB-4), available for $4 from the Canadian Wood Council, 55 Metcalfe, Ottawa K1P 6L5.

FRUITWOOD

I have a piece of furniture that I am told is made of fruitwood. What is this, exactly?

It is simply wood from a fruit tree. European fruitwood is generally pear. In North America apple and cherry are also used, although the latter usually goes by its own name.

HEATING VALUE OF WOOD

We have a convenient source of firewood at a very reasonable price and are thinking of adding a wood-burning unit to our oil furnace. How can we compare the cost of the two fuels?

The heat energy in wood varies according to its weight, species and moisture content, but a cord of most air-dried hardwoods burned in a wood furnace is roughly equivalent to 460 litres of fuel oil. If you want to compare other furnace fuels, a cord of firewood would be equal to 530 cubic metres of natural gas or 3000 kilowatt-hours of electric heat.

LOG SLICE TABLETOP

I have cut a 3 in. slice of a maple log 20 in. in diameter and would like to make this into a table top. How can I keep it from splitting, and what finish should I use to retain the natural color of the wood?

There are chemical treatments that will prevent green wood from shrinking and cracking as it dries out, but it's not practical to undertake such a project yourself and I don't know of any company that will do it for you.

All the tables you see made of log rounds have a number of radial cracks, but they are filled very skillfully with special materials mixed to match the color of the wood. You can buy plastic-based wood fillers that will do much the same job at any hardware store. Wrapping the green wood in burlap to keep it from drying out too quickly will help to reduce the cracking.

Any of the transparent wood finishes will preserve the natural wood color as long as the table is not left outdoors, although there will always be some darkening with age. I suggest either a clear lacquer or four coats of satin urethane varnish, wet-sanded between coats.

PITCH POCKETS

Last spring we had a pressure-treated wood deck added to the back of our house. As soon as the hot weather came, sticky sap began to ooze out of cracks in the wood. As fast as we could scrape it off, more would come out. How can we correct this problem?

That must have been very poor quality wood, but it probably won't do much good to complain about it now. The problem is caused by pitch pockets in the wood expanding as they are heated. The only remedy is to open the pitch pockets with a chisel, scrape out as much of the pitch as you can, then flush out the rest with petroleum solvent. Fill the holes with plastic wood and stain this to match the rest of the deck.

BURNING PRESSURE-TREATED LUMBER

I used pressure-treated lumber to build some fences and a large deck last summer and saved the scraps to burn in my fireplace. Now someone has told me this can be dangerous. Is that true?

The green-colored chemicals used in most pressure-treated lumber have a copper arsenate base. While the treated wood itself is not considered harmful to humans, animals or vegetation, the Canadian Institute of Treated Wood says that burning such wood in a fireplace could release hazardous chemicals into the air. The risk is slight, certainly, but caution would be advisable, particularly if you have a lot of such lumber to dispose of. CITW recommends that it be buried in a sanitary land fill site.

PRESSURE-TREATED PILES

Soil tests on our building lot have indicated that we need to have piles driven in the ground to support the foundation of a new house. Pressure-treated wooden piles would be a lot cheaper than steel piles, we are told, but we are concerned that these might rot.

Neither steel nor treated wood will last forever, but wooden piles that are impregnated with preservative chemicals up to the CSA standard required for wood foundations will last at least as long as the rest of the house. This standard calls for .6 pounds of preservative per cubic foot, compared to the .4 pounds per cubic foot normally used for pressure-treated outdoor lumber. You should obtain the treated piles from a company that is certified by CSA to produce the lumber used for preserved wood foundations. And since the weight of a concrete foundation might be a problem in the type of construction you are considering, I suggest that you consider using preserved wood foundations instead. Talk to your builder about it.

WATER STAINS ON WOOD

Water leaked in on our basement floor and soaked the bottom of the cedar panelling in one corner. This has left a flame-shaped pattern of brown water stains on the unfinished wood. Is there anything we can use to get rid of these?

Because the wood pigments are soluable in water, they can be removed by rubbing the stain area with a moist cloth to which a few drops of sink detergent have been added. When the stain has gone, wring out the cloth and wipe the wood around the area to prevent other water rings from forming. A moderate-strength solution of chlorine laundry bleach will also work – say, one part to five parts water.

WOOD FINISHING

CEDAR SIDING NATURAL FINISH

We have built a holiday cottage with rough cedar siding that is presently unfinished. We know that this wood weathers to a silvery grey color that many people find attractive, but we would rather keep the cedar in its present reddish brown color. What finish should we apply to do this?

The usual recommendation is to apply a pigmented stain in the shade you want, and this is still good advice. But I have recently learned of a treatment that was developed by the California Redwood Association to retain the natural color of that wood, which is very close to the color of our Western red cedar. The treatment is not a finish, in the usual sense, but a water-repellent preservative that reduces color changes due to weathering, water staining and mildew growth, all of which contribute to the grey color of aged cedar.

The solution consists of 3½ cups of pentachlorophenol wood preservative (5%); 1½ cups of boiled linseed oil; 1 ounce of paraffin wax (melted), and 2 quarts of petroleum solvent or paint thinner. (If you prefer metric, use 800ml of pentachlorophenol wood preservative (5%); 350ml of boiled linseed oil; 30ml of paraffin wax (melted), and 2.6 litres of petroleum solvent or paint thinner.)

Applied generously, one gallon will do about 200 square feet of rough cedar or 400 square feet of smooth cedar. (One litre will do 4 square metres or 8 square metres, respectively.)

If the wood starts to show blotchy discoloration after the first year, scrub it gently with a mild detergent solution, rinse, dry, and then make another generous application of the wood preservative solution. The second treatment should last much longer.

FINISHING CEDAR PANELLING

I have purchased a home with a completely finished basement that is panelled with tongue-and-groove cedar. This does not appear to have any finish on it at all. Is there something I should put on to maintain the natural color?

I have seen a great many architect-designed homes with interior panelling in cedar, and in almost all cases it has been left completely natural, with no finish or other treatment at all. That is the way I have used it in my home, too. Anything you put on it will change the color to some extent, and mask the pleasant odor of the wood.

FINISHING CEDAR PATIO FURNITURE

I am building a circular picnic table and four curved benches out of red cedar, and want to be able to keep them outside all year. I would like to apply a smooth, water-clear finish that will be easy to keep clean and will not become dull or crack and peel with outdoor exposure so it has to be refinished every couple of years. I have seen a finish like this on picnic tables in some of our provincial parks.

The government parks department would also like to find such a finish. They have to take benches and picnic tables into the maintenance shops every fall to be stripped and refinished with several coats of varnish. There is no clear film finish that will last outdoors for more than a few years in our climate. The most durable finish tested by the National Research Council is four coats of a standard phenolic varnish, usually sold as marine or spar varnish. (Urethane is not recommended for exterior use.) But even this should be recoated as soon as the surface begins to get dull.

In my opinion, the best finish for cedar garden furniture is no finish at all, but a tabletop will be easier to keep clean if it is sealed with two coats of a penetrating oil/resin finish that you can make with one part spar varnish, two parts boiled linseed oil and three parts petroleum solvent (Varsol etc.). Brush this on generously, let it stand 15 minutes, then remove all surplus with a dry cloth. Next day, apply a second coat the same way.

CIGARETTE BURNS

I recently bought a secondhand bedroom suite of blonde wood – birch, perhaps – with a shelf headboard that has several cigarette burns on top. Can you tell me how to remove and refinish these?

The burned wood can be removed with a piece of fine sandpaper wrapped around your finger, or with the curved tip of a knife blade used as a scraper. From your description I gather that the wood has not been stained, so when all the discoloration has been removed you can refinish the burn areas with a small brush and two or three coats of clear lacquer. Deeper burns will have to be built up with more coats of lacquer, starting in the centre and applying additional layers until the damaged area is level with the rest of the finish. This won't take too long because lacquer dries very quickly and can be recoated in about 20 minutes. If this work is done carefully, the damaged area will be almost invisible.

CIGARETTE BURN ON FINE TABLE

My fine old mahogany dining table recently received a deep cigarette burn in a very conspicuous spot. Is there any way I can repair this myself, or do I have to have the table completely refinished?

No to both questions. It takes special materials and a lot of skill to restore damage like this invisibly in a valuable table, but there are experts around who can do it without refinishing the entire top. Furniture stores hire them to repair scratches, dents and other damage caused during shipment or handling. Ask a store that specializes in fine furniture to give you the name of someone who does this work, or look in the Yellow Pages under Furniture Repairing & Refinishing.

DANISH OIL FORMULA

I have an early copy of your book, *Easy Furniture Finishing*, in which you gave a formula for making a penetrating oil/resin or Danish oil finish for furniture. This called for one part boiled linseed oil, one part varnish and one part turpentine. Regular varnish is now hard to find; it's all polyurethane now. Will this do?

This is even better. Polyurethane resins are tougher than the phenolic resins that were once widely used in the manufacture of varnishes – and still are to a limited extent, such as for marine use. I would also change the formula slightly: one part polyurethane varnish, two parts boiled linseed oil, and three parts petroleum solvent (Varsol, etc.). The easiest of all finishes, this is simply brushed or wiped on the sanded wood, allowed to sink in for about 15 minutes, then all surplus is removed with a clean, dry cloth. (This step is very important.) A second coat can be applied the same way after 24 hours. The resulting finish is similar in appearance to the one that you see on all teak furniture; the wood retains its natural texture but is sealed to prevent staining and make cleaning easier.

FINISHING A WOOD DECK

Last year I built a wood deck at the back of our house using pressure-treated lumber for the posts but plain lumber for the decking, to which I applied two coats of a cedar-colored stain. By the end of the summer the stain was flaking off in some places and wearing off in others. Should I have put a sealer of some kind over the stain to make it last?

While a stain is fine on vertical surfaces such as siding, I do not recommend using one on a wood deck. Stains are not made to withstand foot traffic, and the pigment that wears off is usually tracked into the house, where it can discolor carpets and even vinyl flooring. Putting a sealer on top of it only delays the problem.

Among other treatments I do *not* recommend are linseed oil, which is slow to dry, collects dust, and encourages mildew; paint, which doesn't wear very well and must be re-done every year or so; and any plastic, varnish or other clear *film finish*, all of which degrade or peel off in time, mainly because sunlight breaks down the surface of the wood and destroys the bond (additives that absorb ultraviolet light will delay this but not prevent it). When a film finish begins to go, it must be stripped off to be re-done, and this is a big job.

A wood deck does not need a "finish" in its usual sense. If it has not been pressure-treated it should just be given a generous application of a clear wood preservative to prevent mildew and algae growth that can discolor the wood. Other than that it should be allowed to weather naturally. All wood turns grey with age, but if you do not like the weathered look you can retard it by applying a penetrating oil/resin sealer such as Watco Exterior Wood Finish, Flecto Varapel or Moorwood Penetrating Clear Wood Finish.

FINISHING CEDAR FURNITURE

I have made a picnic table and some lawn chairs out of cedar. What kind of a finish should I put on them?

Apply one or two coats of a penetrating oil-resin sealer, commonly called Danish oil finish or plastic oil finish. There are several brands on the market. It is simply wiped or brushed on, allowed to sink in for 15 minutes or so, then wiped off with a dry cloth. A second coat can be applied after 12 hours.

LIGHT FINISH FOR WOOD

We are going to panel our living room in white pine, and because the windows only face north we want to keep the panelling as light in color as possible. What is the best finish to use?

Normally, even a colorless clear finish will darken wood to some extent, just as plain water does, and most add an amber tone. There are some little-known lacquer-based sealers that reduce this effect considerably, and also retard the natural yellowing and darkening of wood with age. Three such products are Deft Natural Stain & Tint Base; Fabulon PRYME First Coater & Wood Lightener, and Pratt & Lambert's FILTEX.

If such a sealer is followed by one or more coats of a water-clear lacquer finish, you will have the lightest color that can be obtained with the wood you are using. (Note: lacquers are very inflammable and should only be used in a well ventilated room, away from any open flame.) Lacquers dry very quickly and several coats can be applied in an evening. To be sure you are buying a lacquer, see that the label says to use *lacquer thinner* for dilution and cleanup.

LINSEED, TUNG & TEAK OILS

I have a lot of varnished furniture and would like to know what I should treat it with to maintain a rich sheen. Teak oil, tung oil and linseed oil have all been suggested. How do they compare and what is the proper way to apply them?

Linseed and tung are both "drying oils", which means that they harden on exposure to air, producing a tough, flexible material that makes a good paint film and was also the main ingredient of linoleum. Linseed oil is extracted from the seeds of the flax plant, from which linen is made. The raw oil dries very slowly, so chemicals are usually added to make it dry faster. This is called "boiled" linseed oil, although little or no heat is involved. Tung oil comes from the seeds of the tung tree, native to China, and it's much more expensive than linseed oil. Most authorities find little difference between tung and linseed oil as a furniture finish, but some believe that tung oil is superior.

When used as a furniture finish, tung or linseed oil must be thinned with turpentine or petroleum solvent (mineral spirits) - usually about 50%. The thinned oil is also known as teak oil because it is most commonly used on teak, but it can also be used on walnut, oak and other woods that take an oil finish. It is not meant to be used on furniture with a lacquer or varnish finish, however.

When it is applied to raw or previously oiled wood, the thinned linseed or tung oil should be allowed to sink in for about 15 minutes, *then all surplus must be wiped off with a dry cloth*. If wet oil is left on the surface it will become sticky, collect dust, and ruin the finish.

MATCHING DIFFERENT WOODS

I have an old oak roll-top desk that has been repaired with maple and birch as well as oak. The desk has now been sanded and is ready to be refinished. I want to use a dark stain. What kind of stains should I use to make all three kinds of wood come out the same color?

It's impractical to use different stains to make all the woods match. There should be very little difference, in any case, if you are going to use a dark stain. If necessary, a little more stain can be applied in some areas, or it can be left on the wood a little longer before it is wiped off, in order to arrive at a more even tone.

I suggest using a gel stain, since this is easier to control than conventional oil stains and is less likely to show lap marks. Test the stain in a hidden spot to make sure you have the color you want. Apply as directed, then cover with two or more coats of satin urethane, sanding lightly between coats.

FINISHING PINE FURNITURE

We have just had a very nice kitchen table and chairs made for us in pine. They are unfinished. Would urethane floor varnish make a good, durable finish?

Floor varnishes generally have a high gloss. Satin or semi-gloss urethane makes a better furniture finish. First sand the wood with #180 aluminum oxide paper or #0000 steel wool. Remove the sanding dust, then wipe the wood with a moist cloth and allow it to dry. This will raise any short wood fibres left by the sanding; sand again to remove these and produce a smooth surface ready for finishing. (To see if it's smooth enough, draw a nylon stocking over the surface; if it catches, sand the spot again.) Remove all sanding dust, then apply two or more coats of satin urethane, sanding lightly betwen coats with #300 wet paper.

FINISHING A SAUNA

We have been given various opinions regarding finishing the cedar panelling in our sauna. Doesn't it need a sealer of some kind?

No. The wood should be left unfinished so it can absorb moisture.

STAINING OAK

I am installing a curved staircase with a handrail, balusters and treads of oak. I want to darken the oak a bit, and some Dutch friends tell me that in Holland they do this with ammonia. Does this really work?

That's how "fumed oak" was made. This olive-brown color was originally achieved by sealing oil furniture in an airtight container along with a strong solution of ammonia. The fumes changed the tannic acid in the wood to ammo-

nium tannate, a reddish pigment that produced the distinctive color. You can get the same color by brushing ordinary household ammonia on oak. But ammonia isn't very pleasant to work with, and it may not give you quite the shade you want. I think you would do better to use a regular stain. Try a walnut stain; it looks particularly good on oak.

REMOVING A WOOD STAIN

I am trying to refinish a very old desk that appears to be made of solid birch. I have removed the varnish but even sanding does not remove the reddish-brown stain that I am told was put on with some kind of iodine solution. I want to get back to the natural color of the wood and then apply a clear finish.

None of my reference books, including a very old one on wood finishing formulas, mentions the use of iodine as a wood stain. But if that is what you have, you should be able to remove it with a solution of one tablespoon of sodium thiosulphate (photographer's "hypo", available from any good photo supply store) to 16 ounces of warm water. Most other wood stains, however, can be removed with chlorine laundry bleach, applied full strength. If this is going to work you will see it in the first two or three minutes. Repeat as necessary and rinse thoroughly.

REFINISHING STAIRS

We just bought a 15-year-old, 2-storey house and would like to refinish the hardwood stairs. The varnished wood is scratched in places and there are also some cigarette burns. It would be hard to sand because the railing posts go into the wood. We would like to stain both the stairs and the railing a dark brown. Is this possible?

This is a tedious job but not a difficult one. The best way to remove the finish and get rid of the scratches and burns is with a small belt sander. Start with #40 paper, then go over it again with #80 and end with #120 to get a smooth surface for finishing. With a small sander you should be able to do around the posts, but you may have to use a sanding block (a small block of wood will do very nicely) to get into some places.

It's best to use a chemical paint remover on the handrail and posts, or balusters. Remove the softened varnish with a stiff brush, nylon scouring pad or anything else that works. If you have turned balusters, use a piece of soft rope wrapped with #000 steel wool. A walnut stain looks very good on oak. Follow with two coats of urethane.

URETHANE VARNISH

I sanded and refinished the hardwood floor in our entrance hall, using two coats of a urethane varnish that went on very thin and did not wear very well. I have heard that the quality of urethane varnish depends largely on the amount of urethane it contains, but I cannot find this information on any of the labels, and the sales people in the paint stores say they don't know. Can you tell me where I can get this information?

The durability of urethane varnish does indeed depend to a large extent on the percentage of non-volatile solids (principally polyurethane resin) it contains, and if you were in the United States you would find this printed on every label. But even U.S. brands that are sold here do not carry this information, and there is no regulation in Canada requiring them to do so. There IS a Canadian government standard (#1-GP-175M) that requires a minimum 45% solid content by weight in urethane varnish, but unfortunately this applies only to products purchased by the government, not to products sold to consumers.

There are no industry-wide standards for urethane varnish (or any other paint product) in Canada, and no regulation specifying the minimum amount of polyurethane resin it must contain. The only way you can get this figure is to ask the manufacturer for it, but very few will give it to you. My advice is to buy a brand from one who will. A number of people in the paint business believe that information like this – which has nothing to do with secret formulas, incidentally – should be available to the consumer, and your action might help them convince the industry to do something about it.

APPLYING URETHANE

I have read several times in your column that no more than 24 hours should be allowed between coats of urethane varnish. Why is this?

Urethane is a very tough, durable finish, but it rates low in what paint chemists call "recoatability", meaning that it doesn't stick to itself too well once the previous coat has hardened thoroughly. Most manufacturers specify a time limit of 24 or 36 hours. I use the lower figure to be on the safe side. But even if you want to recoat urethane *after* this time, all you have to do is sand the hardened coat lightly to provide a "tooth" for the next one.

WHAT FINISH IS IT?

I have a solid oak dining table that seems to be losing its finish in some areas. I would like to restore it but I don't know what the finish is. I know it's not shellac because water doesn't turn it white. A friend says it's varnish. I think it may be an oil finish because it soaks up lemon oil furniture polish when I put this on. If it's an oil finish, I'll put on more oil. If not, I would like to apply a satin polyurethane finish. How can I tell?

If it soaks up lemon oil, then it must be an oil finish and can be restored by applying one of the Danish oil finishes (Watco, Rez, Sheffield) with a pad of #0000 steel wool. Note that this must be wiped off with a dry cloth after 15 minutes or so. Do not let the wet film dry on the surface. A second coat can be applied the next day, if desired.

Urethane can be applied over an oil finish or varnish, but not over lacquer or shellac. You can test for this in an inconspicuous spot with a cloth moistened with lacquer thinner. If this removes the finish, it's lacquer. Lacquer thinner will not affect varnish.

MISCELLANEOUS

ACID DISCOLORS STONE

I recently purchased a new home and attempted to remove mortar stains from the stone veneer facing with muriatic acid. I diluted it a bit, but apparently not enough because it has turned the grey stone a nicotine color. I have tried a number of cleaning solutions with negligible results. How can I get rid of this stain?

The standard commercial grade of muriatic acid should not be used on stone, brick or concrete any stronger than one part to 10 parts water, in spite of the instructions you may read on the label of some brands. The stain you have on the stone is called "acid burn", and it can be removed with a strong solution of oxalic acid crystals. You can get these from any druggist; it may even be on the store shelves labelled as Rust Remover. There is also a brand of oxalic acid rust remover called ZUD, which is available at most supermarkets. Soak a piece of cloth in a concentrated solution of the crystals and place it on the stain.

ALUMINUM POT BLACKENED

Can you tell me how to clean an aluminum saucepan that has turned black on the inside because of something that was boiled in it?

A steel wool soap pad will remove the tarnish, but an easier way to do it is to fill the saucepan with water above the tarnish line, bring it to a boil and add a heaping teaspoon of cream of tartar, which you probably have among your baking supplies. Continue simmering and the aluminum will become cleaner than you have ever seen it.

ANTS OR TERMITES?

Recently I noticed around our house a large number of flying insects that look like ants. They are black and drop their wings after they land. Could these be termites?

They could be termites or carpenter ants, neither of which is good news around a house. Termites are a much more serious problem, however. They have two pairs of paddle-shaped wings of equal length, while ants have back wings that are shorter then the front ones. But the easiest way to distinguish them is by the difference in the shape of their bodies. Termites have a one-piece, pear-shaped body, while ants' bodies are in two distinct sections.

BENDING ARBORITE COUNTERTOP

I would like to know how to bend Arborite so I can curve it up the back of my kitchen counter.

A special "forming" grade of Arborite that can be softened by heat is used for this purpose, and special equipment is also needed. The standard grade of Arborite cannot be softened by heat. You'll have to use it flat, and make the back of the counter out of a separate piece.

RESTORING WORN COUNTERTOP

The plastic countertop in our kitchen is beginning to show signs of wear after 15 years. The surface is no longer shiny in some places and the pattern is disappearing in areas that get a lot of use. Is there any way I can restore this?

The melamine wear layer on plastic laminate countertops like Arborite and Formica is a very tough and durable material, but it *does* wear through in time, exposing the more delicate patterned paper surface underneath. When this becomes worn there is no way to restore it; all you can do is replace the laminate top. If the counter has a square front edge and the laminate is well attached, it can simply be sanded lightly and then covered with new laminate applied with contact cement. But if the countertop has a rolled front edge and a coved, integral splashback, you will have to replace the entire countertop.

BARBECUE CORRODED

A white, powdery corrosion has formed on our outdoor gas barbecue unit, particularly on the bottom and around the draft intake slots. How can I remove this and prevent it from recurring?

Cast aluminum barbecue units are often made of low quality, reclaimed metal that contains impurities such as copper and iron that promote corrosion from air-borne acids and other pollutants. While the corrosion does not look very nice, it does not affect the performance or durability of the unit. It can be removed with coarse steel wool or a wire bursh. Then use a matt black, high temperature paint, available at any auto supply store, to restore the finish. The paint will also help to prevent further corrosion.

BARN SWALLOWS

Every spring our country house is plagued by barn swallows that build nests under the eaves and generally make a mess of things. I knock the nests down each fall but that doesn't keep the swallows from coming back. How can I discourage them?

There's no guaranteed method but I can suggest a couple of tricks that sometimes work. One is to hang strips of aluminum foil from the edge of the roof. These should be long enough to blow around a bit in the breeze. I've also been told that those little plastic windmills-on-a-stick they sell at circuses and fairs (and probably toy stores, too) will often keep birds away. You could tack a few of these along the edge of the roof, as well.

APPLYING BATHTUB CAULK

I have never been able to make a neat job of applying caulking compound around our bathtub. It always ends up smeared and lumpy. What is the trick?

The best trick I know of is to apply a strip of masking tape to both the tub and the wall, about a quarter of an inch out from the joint. Squeeze a bead of caulking compound along the joint, *pushing* the nozzle instead of pulling it as most people do, to force the caulking compound into the corner. Then spread the sealant with a moistened finger to create a smoothly coved joint. Remove the two strips of masking tape before the caulking begins to harden.

You will have to remove the old caulking compound before you start this job, of course. The best way to do this is with a razor-blade scraper, the kind used for removing paint from windows. (There is no solvent for silicone caulking compound.) Wash the wall and tub surfaces to remove any soap film, then allow them to dry completely before applying new caulking as described above.

POLISHING A FIBREGLASS BATHTUB

We have a molded fibreglass bathtub and shower unit that is very comfortable and attractive. The only problem is that the shine has started to wear off in places. It would cost $800 to have a new finish put on. Isn't there a way we can repolish it ourselves?

The wear surface of your fibreglass tub/shower unit is either an acrylic plastic or a polyester-styrene gelcoat. Both of these materials can be repolished with ordinary brass or silver polish on a soft cloth. A lambswool buffing pad on an electric drill will do the job a lot faster but this must be used very cautiously on an acrylic surface because the plastic can be softened or even melted by the heat of friction if you press too long or too hard in one place. However you do it, the job takes patience, but it does work.

BATS IN THE ATTIC

Can you tell us how to get rid of the bats that have taken up residence in our attic?

They can sometimes be driven out by sprinkling a generous amount of moth crystals around the attic. Three to five pounds of paradichlorobenzine, available at any drug store, will do the average attic. But a simple, cheap, humane way to chase bats away is to keep a light burning up there for 24 hours a day during the summer months. Bats don't like light.

As soon as the bats have gone, cover all possible entry holes with galvanized metal sheets of 1/4 in. mesh screen. (They will usually leave the attic before winter comes, in any case, in order to go into underground hibernation.)

STORING BATTERIES

Is it possible to increase the shelf life of flashlight batteries by storing them in the refrigerator?

This should not be done with the alkaline batteries that are now very common, but it does work on the cheaper zinc-carbon batteries. The storage life of these is about one year, but it can be doubled by keeping them in a refrigerator – or better still, in a freezer. The batteries must be kept in a vapor-tight plastic bag, however, to prevent condensation forming on them. They should be taken out of the fridge a few hours before they are to be used so they can warm up to room temperature.

Alkaline drycell batteries should be kept in a moderately cool place, such as the basement, but should NOT be refrigerated. This also applies to the small mercury, silver or lithium button cells used in watches, hearing aids, etc.

CEDAR PANELLING IN BATHROOM

We want to re-do our bathroom and are thinking of panelling it entirely with tongue-and-groove cedar in a diagonal pattern. What is the best way to apply this, and how should it be finished?

Cedar is a beautiful wood but I do not recommend putting it around the tub/shower enclosure because there is no way to seal the joints between the boards. A plastic laminate such as Arborite or Formica or one of the 3-piece moulded plastic "tub surrounders" would be much better here.

You can nail the cedar panelling to the walls if you locate the studs first and mark their position with pencil or chalk lines, then drive 1½ in. finishing nails through the tongue of the V-joint at an angle. I have found it works better, however, to apply the strips of panelling to the wall with dabs of mastic adhesive spaced about 2 ft apart, and use nails only where needed to hold a warped board to the wall while the adhesive sets.

The diagonal pattern is easy to do if you start in a lower corner with a triangular piece of panelling with the tongue facing up. The length of this becomes the smaller length of the next piece, with 45° cuts at each end. You will soon work out a system to measure, cut and fit the boards as you go along. The diagonal pattern will look best if the boards on adjoining walls coincide exactly to form 90° chevron stripes. Start in any lower corner, but follow this zig-zag pattern as you work around the room.

There are two schools of thought about finishing cedar. I prefer no finish at all. This retains the natural color and pleasant smell of the cedar. The odd splash of water will not mark the wood, and any blemishes that do appear can be sanded off quite easily. Others prefer a finish that can be wiped clean. The most natural finish is a penetrating oil/resin treatment that is usually called a Danish oil finish or plastic oil finish. This darkens the wood slightly (about as much as wetting it with water) but retains its natural texture. It is simply brushed on, allowed to sink in for 15 minutes or so, *then wiped off.* Two applications should be given. For a really scrubbable finish, use two or more coats of satin urethane. But I still recommend leaving it alone; you can always finish it later if you change your mind.

DISCOURAGING BIRDS

We are having trouble with birds parking on our eavestroughs and messing up the front of our house. How can we stop them doing this?

I know someone who stopped this problem by applying white grease along the edge of his eavestroughs. He tied a piece of cloth around the end of a long stick and used this to apply the grease. It's worth a try.

CENTIPEDES IN THE HOUSE

I have been finishing my basement and have found a number of centipedes, both dead and alive, around the area. I am puzzled as to how they get in and would like to know how to get rid of them.

There are lots of cracks in the framework of a house that are big enough for an insect to get through – around the doors and windows, for instance, or over the top of the foundation wall. But think twice about getting rid of all the centipedes. They are classified as a beneficial insect because they prey on destructive insects and do no harm themselves. The removal of dark hiding places around the outside of the house, such as boards, leaves and firewood, will help to reduce their population, however.

CUTTING ARBORITE

I have made some small tables that I want to cover with Arborite or Formica, but I am not able to saw this material without chipping the edges. What is the trick?

There are several tricks for cutting plastic laminate. One is to use a fine-toothed saw. The common handsaw usually has eight teeth to the inch, referred to as an 8-point saw. A 12-point saw is recommended. The laminate should be firmly supported on both sides of the cut, and the saw should be held at a low angle of about 30°. Cut only on the downstroke; don't apply any cutting pressure on the upstroke. Another trick is to cover the cutting line with transparent tape.

If you are using a portable power saw, either circular or sabre, the decorative face of the laminate should be on the bottom, since both of these saws cut on the upstroke. Again, a fine-tooth blade should be used. If you use a table saw, which cuts on the downstroke, the decorative face should be on top.

For straight cuts, however, the easiest way to cut this material is to scribe it with a special plastic laminate scoring tool and then snap it off over the corner of a table or other firm support. Some chipping may still occur, however, and most authorities recommend cutting all pieces about 1/8 in. (3mm) oversize, then trimming the excess off later with a router, block plane or file. This also assures a better fit.

CLEANING BONE HANDLES

I would like to know how to clean the bone handles on a set of old English cutlery.

Use a mild bleach such as hydrogen peroxide and ammonia, or lemon juice and salt. Wet a cotton pad with the peroxide and add a few drops of household ammonia, then rub on the bone handles. For the lemon juice treatment, put some in a saucer, sprinkle with salt, then dip a cotton pad in the solution.

CLEANING A RANGE HOOD FILTER

What is the best way to clean the aluminum mesh grease filter in the vent hood over my stove?

Use a spray-on degreasing solvent such as Polyclens, Gunk or Dunk, sold at most hardware and auto supply stores. Allow this to sink in for a few minutes, then rinse off under the laundry tub taps, or take it outside and use a hose. Repeat if necessary.

A COLD CELLAR THAT ISN'T

We bought a house last year that has a cold storage room in the basement. It has a tight-fitting door, seems to be well insulated, and is cold enough in winter. It doesn't seem to be cold at all in the late spring and summer, however. Please tell me what I can do to keep my cold cellar cold.

I think you're expecting too much of a cold cellar, which is really meant for the *winter* storage of fruits and vegetables, keeping them just above the freezing point. In summer it should still be the coolest room in the house, but at best it will always be a little warmer than the earth outside the walls, probably no cooler than 16°C (60°F). If you want it colder than that you will have to put in refrigeration equipment.

BE YOUR OWN CONTRACTOR?

Is it true that I can build my house a lot cheaper by acting as my own contractor?

Only if you've had a lot of experience in house building. Otherwise I don't recommend it. About 40 different trades are involved in building a house, and getting all of this work done correctly and at the right time is a full-time job even for an experienced contractor. If subtrades don't turn up when they're supposed to, you will have to pay other workmen to stand around and wait. And if they don't do a job the way you wanted it, what pressure can you use to get them to correct it? You're not going to hire them again, anyway. As an owner-contractor, you may also have some difficulty getting a mortgage, building permits, insurance and warranty coverage.

And for all the work and worry, chances are that you won't save any money. You will pay more for materials and subtrades than an established contractor does, and run up a lot of other expenses because of lack of experience. There are other problems, but these should be enough to convince you that being your own contractor isn't a very good idea.

The best thing to do is ask several well-established builders to bid on your specifications and plans. I'd be willing to bet that the lowest price would be no more, and probably less, than it would cost you if you were your own contractor.

COPPER CLEANER

I was given a large, antique copper boiler that is solid black with tarnish. What is the best way to restore the copper and keep it shiny?

There are a number of very good copper cleaners on the market, but you can make your own by mixing equal parts of salt and flour and adding enough vinegar to make a paste that can be spread on the tarnished boiler. You will find that it works best if you do one small area at a time. The paste will remove the black tarnish very quickly but it leaves the copper a dull reddish color. To bring up the bright metal, rub it with #0000 steel wool. Remove all finger marks with a soft cloth, then apply a protective coating of clear lacquer with a brush or spray can.

MUST A COPPER POT BE LINED?

I use a set of copper pots for cooking, and one of them, a large frying pan, is beginning to lose the silver coating inside. The copper is now showing through in places. Is this dangerous?

Not if you keep the copper clean and do not cook highly acidic foods in it, according to Dr. Herbert Scheinberg of the Albert Einstein College of Medicine in New York, a leading authority on copper toxicity. Acidic foods include lemon juice, vinegar, sauerkraut, dried fruits, sweet-and-sour sauces and anything cooked in wine.

A plain copper cooking utensil is not poisonous in itself, however. Candy manufacturers and brewers have been using them for years. Our bodies require a small amount of copper, anyway, and are equipped to get rid of a moderate surplus before it does any harm. Highly acidic foods, however, can dissolve enough copper to spoil the taste of the food and perhaps even upset your stomach. And the green corrosion salts that sometimes form on the surface of copper can make you sicker, because they dissolve more easily. This does not mean that copper is a poison in the usual sense, however. Dr. Michael McGuigan, toxicologist at the Toronto Hospital for Sick Children, points out that copper sulphate was once commonly prescribed as an emetic. But Dr. McGuigan has seen no cases of poisoning from using copper cooking utensils.

Copper utensils are lined with a very thin layer of tin or nickel to make them easier to keep clean and prevent chemical reactions that could taint the food and perhaps upset someone who ate it. Such a coating does not affect copper's biggest advantage in cooking – its ability to conduct heat rapidly and evenly over the entire cooking surface. So although there is very little risk in using a copper pan with a worn coating, provided you do it carefully, it is certainly advisable to have it recoated. To find someone in your area who does this work, check the Yellow Pages under *Tinning* or enquire at a store dealing in restaurant equipment.

REMOVING CORK WALL TILES

We just moved into a house with dark cork tiles on the living room wall. They have been applied with contact cement, and I would like to know how to remove them without damaging the wall, which we would like to cover with wallpaper.

Your walls are probably panelled with gypsumboard, and there is no way to get the tiles and contact cement off this without damaging the paper face on the panelling. The best remedy is to leave the tiles there and apply a new layer of gypsumboard on top of them, using panel adhesive. (Exterior corners should be reinforced with metal bead.) When the joints are taped and filled you will have a smooth new wall surface ready for painting or papering.

COUNTERTOP SCORCHED

I accidentally scorched the matt surface of my kitchen countertop, which I believe is plastic laminate. It is only a slight discoloration, but very noticeable. Can you tell me how to remove it?

Hydrogen peroxide will sometimes remove a scorch stain. Use it full strength and add a few drops of household ammonia to start the action. If this doesn't work, try fine steel wool (#0000), which will not mar the matt finish. If the burn is deeper than the paper-thin melamine surface coating, however, there will be no way to remove it.

RECOATING DISHWASHER RACKS

The plastic coating has come off the wire racks in my dishwasher and the metal is beginning to rust. Is there a material I can use to patch the plastic coating?

You can patch it with a general purpose white silicone caulking compound. DO NOT USE BATHTUB CAULK. (This contains a poisonous fungicide that is added to prevent mildew.)

Clean the exposed metal with steel wool, wipe clean, then squeeze a little of the caulking compound on the bare wire and spread it with a moistened finger. Allow it to set for 24 hours before using the dishwasher.

KEEPING DOCUMENTS DRY

I have a small safe in the basement that I keep some documents in, but they get damp. I believe there is a compound of some kind I can put in the safe to absorb moisture and keep the papers dry. Can you tell me what this is?

The product you want is silica gel, which is capable of absorbing up to half its weight in water. It is a white, granular powder that looks like sugar and is often packed in small envelopes along with products that can be damaged by moisture, such as cameras, binoculars, etc. You must have thrown away dozens of them. Silica gel is not easy to find on the retail market, however, although some garden stores and hobby shops sell it for drying flowers. Chemical supply companies also carry it. All you need is a couple of ounces to put in a small cloth bag or a jar with a perforated cap. When you find that it is no longer absorbing moisture, just put it in the oven at 200°F for about 30 minutes. (Some silica gel includes crystals of an indicator chemical that turns blue when the gel is saturated.)

DRYWALL JOINTS BUBBLING

Two summers ago I applied new gypsumboard panelling over a textured plywood wall, being careful not to overlap the same joints. The new joints were filled with spackling compound, taped, and then covered with two more coats of the filler. Now all the joints have cracked and some of them have bubbled. Can you tell me what I did wrong and how I can fix it?

The bubbles are caused by a poor bond between the joint compound and the tape, probably because the first taping coat of joint compound wasn't allowed to dry properly before the next coat was applied. You may also have used the wrong material to fill the joints. Spackling compound is not the same as drywall joint compound. It is meant for filling cracks and small holes, but sets up too quickly to be used to fill large, deep gaps and does not contain the reinforcing fibres needed to strengthen drywall joints and give them a little flexibility.

The best you can do now is remove all the loose compound and tape and then refill the joints with drywall compound (and new tape, where necessary), feathering it out wider then the original filler.

DRYWALLING OVER OLD PLASTER

I recently purchased an old 2-storey home with lath-and-plaster walls that are badly cracked. I have been told that I must remove all the plaster in order to put up gypsumboard drywall panelling. I would like to avoid that dirty job and simply apply the drywall directly over the plaster. Can I do that?

If the plaster is reasonably smooth and level, or can be made so by removing some of the loose plaster, you can simply glue the gypsumboard directly to it with drywall adhesive applied to the back of the panel with a notched trowel. Use nails along the top and bottom of the wall to hold the panels in place while the adhesive is drying (usually 48 hours), then fill, tape and sand the joints as usual. This is a standard method of drywall application.

If the plaster wall is not level enough to permit this, apply horizontal 1x2 or 1x3 strapping to the wall and insert wood shims behind it to achieve a level surface, then screw the gypsumboard panels to the strapping.

FENCES AND PROPERTY LINES

A group of us at a house party got to talking about fences and property lines the other night, and it soon became apparent that nobody was very sure about where the fence is supposed to go, which way it should face, who pays for it, who maintains it or who has the right to change it. Can you give us the answers?

Most municipalities have a bylaw that covers these questions, but some are more detailed than others. Ask your local building department or public works department for a copy of their fence regulations.

The general rule is that a common fence should straddle the property line, with the posts on one side and the facing material on the other. Minimum construction specifications will be given - generally a galvanized, chain-link fence with posts no more than 10 ft apart extending 3 ft into the ground. The maximum height is also specified. The cost of erecting and maintaining the common fence is shared by both owners. If your neighbor wants a more expensive fence than you are willing to pay for, you need only agree to pay an amount equal to your share of the minimum fence required. Your neighbor must pay the rest. He would also have to pay the same share of any repairs that are required.

If you and your neighbor are unable to agree on the type of fence to put up, the problem can be submitted to an arbitration board, which will probably decide on the minimum fence described in the bylaw.

If your neighbor puts up a fence you don't like, without your approval, and refuses to change it, you can lodge a complaint with the municipal department in charge. They will investigate and recommend further action, if required, but this process can take a long time. The only other option is to build another fence on your side of the property line, but you must leave enough room for repair work to the existing fence - 8 in. is usually considered sufficient.

Neither party has the right to take a property line fence down or change it in any way without approval of the other owner. This applies to subsequent owners, as well.

Another common problem is the case of the vacant lot where adjoining property owners have already built the fences. The law usually specifies that whoever buys and builds on the vacant lot must pay the neighbors a fair share of the cost of building the existing fences.

DOG MOVED OUT, FLEAS REMAIN

We bought our first house a year ago. The previous owner had a dog, and since then we have noticed fleas in the house periodically. We do not own a pet of any kind. Is it possible that the fleas could have survived this long? More important, we would like to know how to get rid of them because we have a six-month-old baby.

Fleas can survive up to a year without food (blood), but will turn to humans if their preferred host such as a dog or cat is not available. So either these are not fleas, or you and your wife - and probably the baby, too - must have been bitten many times in the past year. (Adults generally get bitten on the ankle, and usually in a straight line, curiously enough.) I cannot believe that you would not have noticed these bites. As further identification, fleas range from $1/16$ to $1/8$ in. (2mm to 3mm) in length and are flattened from side to side. Their most distinctive feature, however, is that they can jump about 6 in. high and 16 in. horizontally (150mm, 400mm). If your insects don't jump like this, they are not fleas.

A thorough, frequent vacuuming will gradually get rid of the eggs, pre-adult pupae in hard-shelled cocoons, and adult fleas. Put a handfull of mothballs or moth flakes in the vacuum cleaner bag first, however, to kill anything that is picked up. With a crawling baby in the house, the use of an insecticide spray is not recommended, but if the problem continues you can hire a pest control expert to apply an approved spray while you are away from the house long enough for it to dry completely before you return. Even then the baby should be kept off the floor for a couple of weeks. All approved insecticides will degrade and become harmless in that time.

FROST IN THE ATTIC

Three years ago we had fibreglass insulation blown into the attic of our 2-storey home. We also had the roof reshingled and four vents put in it. Ever since then, frost has formed in our attic during cold weather and dripped on our ceiling when the temperature warms. Now we must have the ceiling repaired, but I want to find a remedy for the problem first. We had no trouble before the ceiling was insulated.

I suspect that the fibreglass wool was blown in to the very edge of the roof, where the rafters overhang the ceiling, and this has blocked the ventilation from the eaves. As a result, you now have less ventilation in the attic than you had before. Someone will have to go up there and rake the fibreglass away from the edge of the roof, leaving space for ventilation between the bottom of the rafters. You can get special plastic or cardboard chutes that will keep these vent spaces open. Large mailing tubes can also be used.

FROST DAMAGE TO FOUNDATION

Our cottage is located in a very cold area and we keep a little heat on all winter to prevent frost damage, although we only use it occasionally. I am still worried about possible frost damage to the foundation walls, however, and would like to know whether I should insulate them to prevent this from happening.

Insulating the foundation walls will keep the cottage warmer, but it increases the chance of structural damage due to frost heave because it allows the frost to penetrate deeper outside the walls.

Studies by the National Research Council's Divison of Building Research in Saskatoon have shown that frost damage to foundation walls can be prevented by laying polystyrene foamboard insulation on the ground three to 6 ft out from the house. This should be at least 2 in. thick, preferably twice that, and covered with concrete paving slabs or earth to hold it in place and shield it from sunlight.

The layer of insulation on the surface of the ground greatly reduces frost penetration and the risk of damage to the foundation walls.

FROST LIFTS VERANDA

Every winter the veranda on the front of our house is lifted by frost heave. I thought I'd fixed it when I dug out the clay soil to a depth of 5 ft and poured round concrete piers to support the framework, but last winter it shifted again when the new piers lifted. I'd like to fix it properly this summer. Can you tell me how to do it?

Normally, piers extending below the frost level will not be moved when the soil freezes. But if the soil is very wet a phenomenon called "adfreezing" can bond the frozen earth to the concrete so firmly that the post will be lifted with the heaving soil. Improving the drainage will help to prevent this. So will anchoring the pier to a footing slab at least twice as wide as the pier.

Both of these involve a lot of work. An easier trick that sometimes works is to dig a funnel-shaped depression around the pier and pour in some old motor oil. The object is to coat the sides of the concrete pier with oil so the soil won't stick to it. This trick is used to keep telephone poles from being lifted by frost heave, I am told.

GLUING CLEAR PLASTIC

I have a cube table made of clear plastic that looks like glass. One of the joints has come apart and I can't find an adhesive that will hold it.

This is probably acrylic, the clearest of the plastics. It is usually connected with welded joints made by using a solvent that dissolves the two surfaces and forms an invisible bond when they are pressed together. Methylene chloride is the solvent, but this is not packaged in small quantities for retail sale. As it happens, however, methylene chloride is also the basic ingredient in paint removers. The thickened ones contain waxes or other chemicals that might weaken the weld, but if you buy one of the water-thin paint removers you will find that this works very well as an acrylic adhesive. Be sure to scrape off any adhesive that is now on the surfaces to be joined. Apply the solvent to both surfaces with a small brush, then press them together and hold them firmly in place with tape for several hours.

REMOVING EPOXY GLUE

I used a 2-part epoxy glue to repair a broken marble statue. It worked fine, but I smeared some of the glue on the surface of the statue and now I can't remove it. What can I use to take this off?

Paint remover will soften epoxy adhesive enough that it can be scrubbed or washed off the marble.

REMOVING KRAZY GLUE

I spilled some Krazy Glue on our plastic laminate countertop and nothing I have tried will remove it. Can you tell me what I should use?

Acetone will dissolve it, but slowly.

FIRMING A GRAVEL PATHWAY

We like the look of the gravel pathways around our house and garden but find the loose gravel very awkward to walk on. Is there something we can put on them, such as cement or crushed limestone, to firm them up?

Crushed limestone makes a very firm paving material by itself, but not if it's mixed with gravel. And you can't just add portland cement to the gravel pathways, either; you would have to remove the gravel and mix it with sand, cement and water in the proper proportions to make concrete, which would then be poured in forms. I don't think this is what you want.

The best way to get the firm, gravel-textured surface you are after would be with "exposed aggregate" concrete. This is made by pouring concrete in the usual way, levelling it with a wood float, and then immediately covering the surface with a layer of gravel or stones that are then pressed into the fresh concrete with a wood float. At this stage the surface will look like conventional concrete, but when the water sheen disappears and the surface is firm enough that thumb pressure will make only a slight impression, a stiff brush and a hose spray is used to remove enough of the sand/cement to expose the top of the gravel or stone layer. This makes a very attractive paving for paths and driveways.

COLORING GLASS

Some years ago we purchased a nice chandelier with amber glass globes. I used to dust these, but recently I decided to wash them. That's when I discovered they were not made of colored glass at all, but just a plastic coating over plain glass. This has now started to peel off. Is there any way I can restore the colored finish?

Many craft and hobby shops sell colored, transparent lacquers that are used for making simulated stained glass windows and other projects. They are often called "glass stains". Use lacquer thinner to remove the old finish.

DECORATING GYPSUMBOARD

We have had an addition put on our house and the drywall panelling has not been finished. How should we prepare this for painting or papering?

If you want to paint the drywall with either a latex or an alkyd or other oil-based paint, apply a latex primer-sealer first. If you want to put up wallpaper, apply an alkyd primer-sealer first.

REMOVING IVY SUCKERS

The front of our house is brick; the sides are covered with white aluminum siding. Some years ago we started growing ivy over the brickwork, and now it has spread over the aluminum side walls. I removed some of this last fall, but the sucker feet have left little black dots on the white siding and I can't seem to get them off. Do you have any suggestions?

Instead of drying up and falling off when they die, as you would expect them to do, the little suckers stick even harder. But if you get at them while they are fresh you will find that they can be taken off quite easily with a bristle brush or a fingernail. If any marks remain on the siding, scrub them off with detergent solution and a nylon scouring pad. The ones that have been there since last fall will have to be scraped off with a knife, but very carefully to avoid scratching the paint.

LAUNDRY TUB LEAKING

I have a crack in my concrete laundry tub that is leaking, and I cannot afford to buy a new one just now. Is there any way I can fix it myself?

A clear silicone caulking compound can be used. Allow the crack to dry thoroughly, then apply the silicone with the tip of your finger to force it into the crack. Wipe off the surplus with a dry cloth and allow the sealer to set for 24 hours before using the tub.

Another filler that can be used is automobile radiator sealer. This should be applied to a wet crack. Simply pour it on, allow it to sink in, then wipe off with a damp cloth.

"BOILED" LINSEED OIL

I have a formula for making an exterior wood stain that calls for boiled linseed oil. I happen to have some raw linseed oil on hand; can I use this instead? If not, can I boil it myself?

Do not attempt to boil linseed oil. The boiling temperature is very high and the oil will smoke badly and may catch on fire before it boils. The term "boiled" is simply a trade expression that refers to a chemical treatment used to speed up the drying time of raw linseed oil. It once involved the use of heat but today it is a cold process, and you can do it yourself just by adding one teaspoon of Japan Dryers to each quart of raw linseed oil. (Most paint stores carry Japan Dryers.) But it won't pay you to do this if you only have a small quantity of raw linseed oil. Besides, linseed deteriorates with age and the old oil may not dry properly. You would be better off to buy new boiled oil.

REPOLISHING MARBLE

I accidentally spilled some vinegar on my polished marble tabletop and it has left a dull spot. Is there any way I can remove this?

The marble has been etched by the acetic acid in the vinegar. (Even soda water is acidic enough to do this.) To repolish this area you will have to rub it with a series of fine abrasives. Start with #320 silicon carbide paper and keep rubbing until there is a very fine, even texture on the stain area, then switch to #400 and do the same. Finish with #600 paper, which should give the marble a soft satin sheen. To achieve a high polish on the marble, rub it with a damp cloth dipped in zinc oxide powder, available from hobby shops that sell rock polishing supplies. Each of these steps takes a lot of rubbing, so be patient. If you rush the job, the etched areas will still have dull spots.

DRAIN CLEANER vs IMITATION MARBLE

We have just had our old-fashioned bathroom sink replaced with an imitation marble vanity/sink combination. Is it safe to use liquid cleaners and cleansing powders on this?

Imitation marble sinks and countertops are coated with a polyester-styrene resin that must meet strict CSA standards for resistance to common household chemicals – incuding a 20%

solution of lye, which is twice as strong as the liquid drain cleaners. But scouring powders should not be used on *any* bathroom sink or tub, according to the fixture manufacturers.

MICROWAVE DOOR SCRATCHED

I used scouring powder to clean the window in my microwave oven door, and it has scratched and dulled the surface very badly. Is there anything I can do to restore it?

The window in most microwave oven doors is made of acrylic plastic that scratches very easily and should not be cleaned with anything but a damp, soft cloth and a drop or two of liquid detergent. The fine scratches that have dulled the surface can be removed, however, by rubbing them firmly with a soft cloth and one of the creamy brass polishes, such as Brasso. Keep rubbing until the surface is shiny smooth. Rinse periodically and blot dry to check your progress.

MILDEW IN CLOTHES CLOSETS

I am having a problem with mildew in our bedroom closets. There is a crawlspace with an earth floor under the bedrooms. I had extra insulation put in the attic and more roof vents added, but this hasn't helped.

The problem is not in your attic. It is due to the condensation of humid household air on the cold walls behind your closets, and there are several things you can do to prevent this. Leaving the closet doors open will help, but this is not very attractive. Laying a sheet of 6-mil polyethylene film over the earth in the crawlspace may also help. But the best remedy is to insulate the outside walls of the closets. All you need to do is cut a sheet of 1 in. thick foamboard into convenient-sized panels and glue them directly to the outside wall. The common white foamboard sold at all building supply stores will do very nicely. Apply a bead of adhesive around the back of each panel, about 1 in. in from the edge, then simply press it in place.

REMOVING MIRROR TILES

I have purchased a condominium apartment that has mirror tiles on the walls. How can I remove these so I can paint the walls?

There is no way to remove the mirror tiles without causing some damage to the face of the gypsumboard wall behind them. The best way to get a smooth, paintable surface is to leave the mirrors where they are and cover them with new gypsumboard panelling applied with adhesive, then fill, tape and sand the joints.

If you really want to remove the mirror tiles, however, you can do it fairly easily if there is an open edge you can get at with a putty knife or a long kitchen spatula. Use this to release the two adhesive pads in the corners of a tile, then pry the edge up gently to pull off the two pads in the back corners. If you do this carefully you won't break a single tile, but it is a good idea to wear leather gloves anyway. If you don't have an exposed edge where you can begin, you will have to break one tile and remove it in pieces to get started. The used tiles can be salvaged by scraping off the old adhesive pads and buying new ones.

MOLD ON SILICONE CAULKING

We used a product labelled as "silicone seal" along the seams of our shower stall. It became coated with mildew so we removed it and applied a new coat of the same material. Shortly thereafter, the mildew reappeared. How can we prevent this?

The compound labelled as "silicone seal" is an excellent general purpose caulking material, but it has a tendency to develop mold in areas where it is exposed to a lot of moisture. The proper silicone to use in this situation is the one labelled "bathtub caulk", which contains a strong fungicide that prevents mold growth.

CLEANING AN OVEN WINDOW

When taking a roast out of the oven I spilled some of the juices on the door. They got in between the two sheets of glass in the oven window and I would like to know how to remove them.

You will have to take the back panel off the door to get at the window, but this only requires removing a few screws. With this out of the way you can remove the metal ring that holds the inside sheet of glass in place so you can lift out the glass and clean it.

PANELLING BUCKLED

Last summer I had insulation and new panelling put in my holiday cottage. I thought they did a wonderful job, but friends who have been watching the unoccupied and unheated cottage for me over the winter tell me that all the walls are buckling. What would cause this?

This sounds like hardboard panelling, which has a tendency to swell when it absorbs moisture. As I'm sure you know, an unheated cottage can get very damp during the winter.

To prevent this problem, the hardboard should have been pre-expanded by wetting the backs of the panels thoroughly about 48 hours before they were put up. Also, a space about the thickness of a penny should have been left between the panels when they were nailed in place. These are the manufacturers' instructions, as a matter of fact, but most builders ignore them.

Unfortunately, the distortion caused by uneven expansion of the hardboard panelling is usually permanent, and the only remedy is to replace it. Gypsumboard or solid wood panelling is less likely to develop this problem.

PATCHING PARGING

The cement plaster or parging on the outside of our foundation wall keeps flaking off. We hired someone to repair it about a year ago, but now it's coming off again, so it couldn't have been done properly. I'd like to try it myself this time. What should I use?

Any concrete patching material or premixed stucco can be used. Available in convenient packages at any hardware or building supply store, these contain acrylic latex bonding agents that provide better adhesion than a straight plaster of portland cement and sand.

Remove all loose material, wet the area to be patched and allow the moisture to sink in before applying the patching material, mixed to a workable consistency. It should be applied at least 1/4 in. (6mm) thick, and finished to match the texture of the rest of the parging. The color will not be the same, however. If the difference is objectionable, paint the wall with any exterior latex paint.

GREEN GROWS THE PATIO

One side of our concrete patio is constantly in the shade, and a green growth has developed there that is both slippery and unattractive. How can I get rid of it?

This algae grows on almost anything that is damp and in the shade, but it grows very slowly. It can be scrubbed off with a stiff brush and a solution of one part chlorine laundry bleach to three parts water plus a heaping tablespoon of *dishwasher* detergent to each quart. (These proportions are not critical; almost any variation of this will do.) You will have to repeat this treatment periodically, however, to keep the patio free of the slippery algae.

PLASTER CEILING SAGGING

I bought an old frame farmhouse with lath and plaster walls and ceilings, which I would like to retain. Unfortunately, parts of the ceiling are sagging and some of the plaster is coming away from the walls, too. Is there any way to re-attach the original plaster to the lath?

There is no way to stick the plaster back again once it has broken away from its support. You might even find that some of the lathing has broken away from the wall, too. You have two choices. One is to find an experienced plasterer to remove the loose plaster and patch the walls. (There aren't many "wet" plasterers around any more.) The other is to nail horizontal 1x3 strapping to the walls – through the plaster and into the studs – and then apply gypsumboard panelling to the strapping. (The ceiling would be done the same way, nailing the strapping to the joists.) When the drywall joints are taped and filled, you will have a new, firm, smooth surface ready for painting or papering.

POLISHING PLEXIGLAS

We have a cube table made of clear Plexiglas. Although we have tried to treat it carefully, the top has been dulled with wear over the years and now looks cloudy. Is there any way we can restore this?

The tiny scratches that have dulled the clear acrylic plastic can be removed by polishing it with a creamy brass or silver polish. Dust it first, then clean the surface with a damp cloth and a couple of drops of dish detergent, making sure no dirt particles that could scratch the plastic are left on the surface. Apply the polish with a soft cloth, rubbing firmly in a circular motion, or use a cloth buffing wheel in an electric drill. Set the drill at a slow speed and don't press too hard or work too long in one spot, however, or the heat of friction will soften the plastic.

Other transparent plastic products, like boat windshields, motorcycle visors and watch crystals can also be repolished with this method.

REPAIRING PORCELAIN ENAMEL

We have mauve-colored bathroom fixtures, and both the bathtub and the basin have small chips that we would like to touch up. The manufacturer tells us this color has not been produced for several years and matching enamel is no longer available. Is there anything else we can use?

Plumbing stores that cater to the home handyman may have some of the old color in stock, or might be able to come fairly close to it. Failing this, you may be able to find a reasonable match in auto body touch-up enamel, which will work just as well. To get a good color match, take along one of the caps that cover the anchor bolts on the base of the toilet. These just pry off.

REFRIGERATOR SCRATCHED

I would like to know if there is any way to remove fine scratches from a refrigerator, made by using scouring powder that is not supposed to scratch.

Scouring powders should not be used on painted surfaces like this, which are generally softer than the finish used on bathroom fixtures and sinks. As a matter of fact, the constant use of scouring powders is not recommended for these, either.

The scratches can be removed with automobile rubbing compound, a gentle abrasive used to smooth auto body finishes, available at all auto supply stores and most hardware stores. Apply the paste with a damp cloth and rub firmly until the scratch marks can no longer be seen. Wash off, dry, and check the finish. If it is slightly dull, apply a coat of paste wax and buff.

RUST FROM WELL WATER

We recently built a house in the country and get our water from a well. It is plentiful, clear and was passed by the health department, but everything it touches becomes stained by rust. The people I've spoken to about this problem all want to sell me something. What is the proper remedy?

The water contains dissolved iron that will stain laundry and affect the taste of many foods. You need a special filter to remove this, but the water should first be tested to determine the amount of iron and hardness chemicals (primarily calcium salts) it contains in order to determine what kind and size of filter you need. Companies that sell water treatment equipment will make these tests for you without charge.

SCOTCH TAPE REMOVAL

My son stuck posters and other pictures to the walls of his room with scotch tape. The walls are hardboard with a printed paper

overlay in a simulated woodgrain pattern. The tape is stuck to the panelling, of course, and will not come off without tearing the paper face.

Lacquer thinner will dissolve the adhesive that holds the tape to the hardboard, and it won't damage the paper face. Moisten a cloth with lacquer thinner and rub the tape patches gently until they peel off.

SPILLED SHELLAC

Last year I built a deck on the back of our house with pressure-treated lumber. This year I accidentally spilled about half a litre of orange shellac on the deck and it has discolored a large area. How can I remove this ugly mark?

Methyl hydrate, available at any hardware store, will dissolve the shellac and soak it into the wood, which should eliminate the stain. Several applications may be necessary, however, to get rid of it completely. Methyl hydrate will not affect the wood preservative, either in color or performance.

DOES GAS BLACKEN SILVER?

We switched our heating system from oil to natural gas a few years ago, and since then it seems that our polished brass and silverware become tarnished much more quickly. Could the gas fuel be causing this?

The association of gas with silver tarnishing goes back to the days when domestic gas was produced from coal and contained a significant amount of sulphur, which is what causes the black tarnish to form on silver, copper and brass. Natural gas does contain a fair amount of sulphur when it comes out of the ground, but this is stripped out, along with other useful chemicals, before it is distributed for use as a heating fuel. Only a few parts per billion remain, and even this is expelled out of the house with the furnace combustion gases, so it really can't be responsible for your tarnished silver.

There are a number of other things that could cause this, however. An increase in local air pollution, such as smoke from a coal-fired generating station, could do it. Another possible cause is an unvented kerosene heater, particularly if this is burning a low grade of kerosene. Even cooking can cause it. Few people realize that a number of common foods contain sulphur and may produce enough hydrogen sulphide when they are cooked to tarnish silver and copper alloys. Cabbage, spinach and rice are particularly bad for this.

SMOKE DAMAGE

We had a bad fire in our house that has left a strong smoke smell in all the clothing and linen. We sent some things to the drycleaner but the odor is still there. How can we get rid of it?

Ordinary drycleaning can set the smoke odor in the fabric. There are firms in every major city that specialize in the restoration of materials that have been damaged by smoke. Unfortunately, the materials they use, which include an ozone generator, are not available on the retail market. Your insurance company can give you the names of firms that do this work – and perhaps they'll pay for it, too. You can also find them listed in the Yellow Pages under Fire Damage Restoration.

REMOVING SOAP FILM

I can't seem to remove the soap film that has formed on the glass doors of our bathtub enclosure. What should I use?

This is probably a combination of soap scum and lime from the water. Wipe it with a cloth soaked in vinegar, doing a small area at a time so the vinegar will have time to dissolve the deposit.

PRESERVING STONE COLOR

I recently had some fieldstone put on the front of my house and was told by the installers that the color of the stone will fade unless we apply a protective coating of linseed oil. Can you give me more information about this?

That is very strange advice indeed. Artificial stone that is colored with pigments will often fade with exposure to sunlight, but the only natural stone I know of that will do this is certain types of limestone. Fieldstone is usually granite, and that will not fade in a million years.

Linseed oil is a poor treatment for stone, in any case. It darkens the color and gives the stone a wet look, certainly, but after a few years this will peel and look very messy. Besides, I assume that it is the color and texture of the stone itself you wanted on your house, and no "protective coating" is required to maintain these.

STONE SIDING

I would like to replace the siding on the front of my house with stone, but I don't want to destroy the garden there by digging it out to put in a foundation to support the masonry. Is there any kind of stone I can put on myself that doesn't need a foundation?

For "veneer" facing like this, stone is available in slabs about half an inch thick. After the siding has been removed, the sheathing and building paper should be covered with metal lath. Cement mortar that contains an acrylic bonding agent is applied to this and the stone slabs are pressed in place.The spaces between the stones can be filled with the same mortar or tuckpointed later with a colored mortar.

This job isn't quite as simple as it sounds, however, and some experience is required to judge the consistency of the mortar and achieve a permanent bond with the stone. I think it should be given to a professional, but ask to see some samples of his work first.

CLEANING STUCCO

Our bungalow is 20 years old and the plain white stucco finish still appears to be in good condition. It is beginning to look a little dingy, however, and I would like to know how it can be freshened up. Is there any way to clean it? Can it be painted? If so, what kind of paint should be used? Does stucco have to be replaced periodically, like shingles?

A good stucco job will last for 50 years or more with a minimum of maintenance. The best way to clean it is with a high-pressure water spray. Equipment for this is available from some tool rental stores. Or use a long-handled stiff brush and a solution of ¼ cup of trisodium phosphate (TSP) to a gallon of water. If you don't want to do the job yourself, look in the Yellow Pages under Building Cleaning - Exterior, for the names of firms that do this work.

Even if you decide to paint the stucco it should be washed first, but a long-handled scrubbing brush and solution of half a cup of trisodium phosphate (TSP) to a pail of water will do the job in this case. Any exterior *latex* paint can be used.

RE-COATING STUCCO

The stucco on our house is in poor condition, and a contractor has offered to apply

a new coat over the existing one. He will apply a bonding coat first, he says, and then put on a rough coat that does not need to be painted. Would that be allright?

Only if the existing stucco is firmly attached everywhere and has never been painted. Stucco will stick to stucco quite well, and a bonding coat will help, but neither can be depended on to hold firmly over an old coat of paint.

REMOVING TAR

We removed a back porch from our old stone house, and this has left a black line of what appears to be tar on the side of the house. How can we remove this?

Tar can be dissolved with lacquer thinner. But it may be asphalt, in which case you can wash it off with Varsol or other petroleum solvent. Try this first; it's a lot cheaper than lacquer thinner. It is a good idea to wear rubber gloves when using such solvents, because they also remove the oils from your skin.

SALT IN WELL WATER

When I purchased my summer home, the well had not been connected to the house yet, but we had the water tested by the provincial health department, and they said it was quite safe for drinking. When I had a chance to taste it, however, I found that it was definitely salty. And it's terrible for washing because it won't make suds at all. Is there anything I can buy that will remove the salt from the water?

Yes. It is known as a reverse osmosis filter, and it is available from firms that sell water softeners. There are small units that can be used to treat drinking water only, or you can get them large enough to de-salt all the water used in the house. Even a small one costs about $500 installed, however.

The water is perfectly safe to drink the way it is, of course, unless there are medical reasons why you must maintain a low-sodium diet. And you can buy special soaps that will lather in salty water.

STATIC PROBLEM

We have a built-in vacuum cleaner and live in a very dusty area. The problem we have is that the long plastic hose of the vacuum cleaner develops a charge of static electricity when it is being used, and this causes it to become covered with dust that rubs off on the clothing of whoever is using it.

Try spraying the vacuum hose with one of the anti-static liquids sold for use on fabrics and carpets.

SUMP PUMP MAINTENANCE

The sump pump in my basement has only operated twice in eight years. When I tried it out recently to see if it was still working, it took several attempts to get it going. What should I do to keep it ready for emergency service?

All mechanical equipment should be operated occasionally to keep it in condition and make sure it will run when needed. You can check the switch and motor just by lifting the float, but a better test is to run a few gallons of water into the sump to make sure the pump and discharge line are also working properly. At the first sign of any difficulty you should have the pump checked and serviced.

THERMOSTAT PROBLEM

Last year I installed a programmable setback thermostat that has a digital time and temperature readout. It also has a rechargeable nicad battery. We were told that this would last for many years, but it went dead during the summer when our hot water heating system was shut off, and had to be replaced. How can we prevent this happening again next summer?

This only occurs with hot water heating systems that have a continuous circulating pump that must be turned off at the end of the heating season. Unfortunately the switch that controls this also supplies the low voltage current to the thermostat that is also used to keep the nicad battery charged. The battery should last a few months even if you turn the power off, but operating instructions for the thermostat usually tell you (in fine print) to leave the power on all year. What they don't tell you is that you may need a separate switch for the pump in order to do this. Homeowners with warm air heating systems will not have this problem; there is no need to turn the power to the furnace off during the summer.

DOES WOOD DUST MEAN TERMITES?

There is a small pile of very fine wood dust at the bottom of a partition wall in our basement. There are also some tiny holes in the wood. Does this mean we have termites?

No. Termites eat the wood; they don't leave any surplus lying around. And they don't make visible entrance holes, either. What you probably do have, however, is a colony of carpenter ants building a nesting gallery inside the framing lumber. Carpenter ants don't eat wood, so they must come out for food, and the best way to eliminate them is to paint a ½% solution of diazinon around all the holes you can see and along the crack at the bottom of the wall. This residual insecticide will be carried back into the nest by the returning workers.

REMOVING WALL ANCHORS

I'm the second owner of a condominium apartment that badly needs redecorating. The former owner apparently had a lot of pictures, because there are a great many of those plastic anchor plugs in the walls. How can I cover or remove these?

Find a screw that fits snugly in the plastic wall plugs. Give it two or three turns, then use a pair of pliers to pull the screw and plug out of the wall. If the paper face of the gypsumboard panelling is frayed around the hole, as it probably will be, cut it back with a razor knife, then use a spatula or putty knife to fill the hole with a plaster patching compound. When this is dry, sand it smooth and apply a second coat of patching compound. A third coat will probably be necessary to get a completely invisible patch. Apply a primer coat to the patches before repainting.

INDEX

122